Possible MIRACLE

A Caregiver's Experience Coping with
Her Husband's Struggle Through
Pancreatic Cancer, Liver Disease
and a Liver Transplant

By Susan Fayne

With Foreword by Charles Miller, MD
Director, Liver Transplantation
Cleveland Clinic

Library of Congress Cataloging-in-Publication Data

Fayne, Susan.
  Possible miracle : a caregiver's experience coping with her husband's struggle through pancreatic cancer, liver disease and a liver transplant / by Susan Fayne.
    pages cm
  ISBN 978-1-62023-115-9 (alk. paper) -- ISBN 1-62023-115-8 (alk. paper) 1. Fayne, Susan. 2. Women caregivers--United States--Biography. 3. Pancreas--Cancer--Patients--Biography. 4. Pancreas--Cancer--Patients--Family relationships--United States. 5. Alpha-1 antitrypsin deficiency--Patients--United States--Biography. 6. Fayne, Michael--Health. I. Title.
  RC280.P25F39 2015
  616.99'4370092--dc23
  [B]
                          2015029362

A miracle cannot prove what is impossible; it is only useful to confirm what is *possible.*

— Maimonides

All proceeds will benefit the

TRANSPLANT HOUSE OF CLEVELAND

Cleveland Clinic is a leader in a variety of transplantation procedures. Their comprehensive life-transforming program has expert physicians and specialists who save thousands of lives every year. Organ transplant is like no other surgery. It affects a family physically, emotionally and financially. Physically, because a patient must be in danger of losing his or her life before they are considered to be placed on a transplant list or be eligible for the surgery. Emotionally, because another person must become a living donor or lose their life for the patient waiting for transplant to survive. Financially, because of the amount of time patient and caregiver need to spend away from their home and job. Above all, the transplant can't be planned for, as the patient never knows exactly when the surgery will take place.

Michael and I were fortunate enough to be able to stay in a hotel for the four months we were in Cleveland before and after his transplant surgery. Many others do not have that ability for various reasons such as family responsibilities, cost, or career related issues. It is so very hard to be away from home, loved ones and friends at a time when you need all of them the most. We both felt how challenging it is to be ill and in a strange city for a long period of time, even though our family was close enough to visit us regularly, so I can't imagine the anxiety and loneliness felt by patients and their caregivers when they must stay close to Cleveland Clinic and are not near anyone or anything familiar.

The Transplant House of Cleveland has been created to help families who have a loved one being evaluated for transplant, waiting for transplant, or recovering from transplant by providing temporary, affordable housing in a home-like environment while in Cleveland for medical care. The newly opened facility provides quality housing in a warm friendly atmosphere at an affordable price. Being with a caring staff, as well as other patients and caregivers supplies great support for those in need. I hope my story will cause readers to recognize the agonizing months transplant patients and their families go through and realize how important it is to aid and assist others who are experiencing the transplant process by offering them the Transplant House as a safe home away from home.

This book is a gift to Cleveland Clinic with all proceeds going to the *Transplant House of Cleveland.*

Please send all donations to: **Transplant House of Cleveland**
2007 E. 115th St. #1 Cleveland, OH 44106
www.transplanthouseofcleveland.org

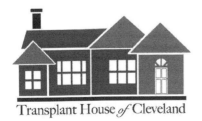

In memory of our dearest Michael Roth

His kindness has touched a countless number of people and will continue to do so even though he is no longer among us. Without his help and encouragement my husband, Michael, would not be here today. Our undeniable gratitude is entrenched in the remembrance of this very special, altruistic man who has given so much to so many.

Possible Miracle

TABLE OF CONTENTS

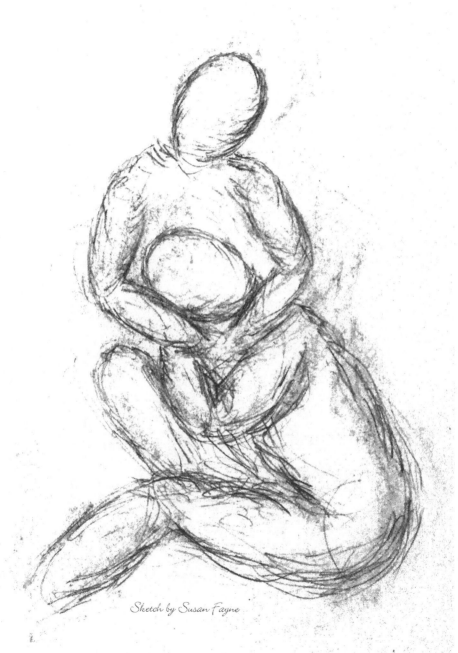

Sketch by Susan Fayne

Possible Miracle

A LETTER TO
MY HUSBAND

To my beloved husband, Michael,

Much of the past year and more has been obscure to you. My desire is that this narrative will make you conscious of the many who worked so hard to save your life and inform you of the events that led them to do so. May we always treasure what they have done for you and the time they have given us.

With love,
Susan

Possible Miracle

A LETTER TO THE READER

My husband, Michael, is a survivor of a savage disease: pancreatic cancer. He has also recovered from a relentless genetic condition, alpha-1 antitripsin deficiency, which severely attacked his liver. He eventually needed a transplant, which he too survived. Together we persevered and lived through those horrendous ordeals; he as a patient and I as a caregiver.

Through each medical condition I lived in a state of denial. Eventually I realized that I had a very sick husband, so I began hoping and praying for him to have a miraculous recovery. Finally I recognized that if I didn't intercede on his behalf and do it quickly, I could lose the man I love. Assuming control and being his advocate saved his life twice. My belief is that my experience will inspire other caregivers to take charge of their own situations and prepare for future problems they may encounter. I have hope that they too can face life's adversities with great fortitude and courage. The most important weapon in a caregiver's arsenal is that of being proactive.

It is also important for the reader to know that the events that happened in our life, in regards to my husband's medical conditions, pertain to his case only. Individuals have different experiences when dealing with cancer, liver disease and especially transplantation. What we went through applies to Michael's particular issues and may not happen similarly in every patient.

If you have chosen to read our book, I trust our path from sickness to health will encourage you.

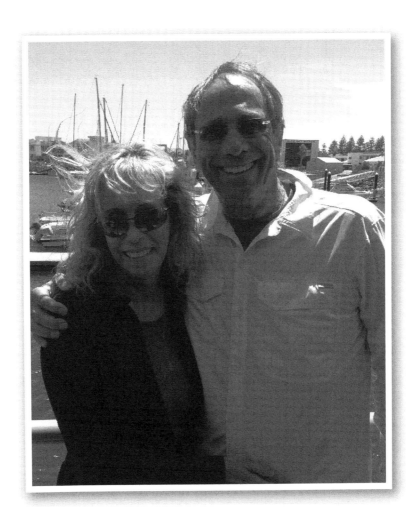

Possible Miracle

ACKNOWLEDGEMENTS

One of the greatest pleasures I have in writing our story is to be able to acknowledge those who have taken part in my husband Michael's care throughout his serious illnesses. I could never properly thank all of them or the institutions that have contributed. It is my desire to show our gratitude by writing this memoir.

Along with Michael Roth, I also dedicate my book to our wonderful children, Amy, Adam and Darren, who are all so uniquely different that they were able to help us in very contrasting ways. Love begins at home and I know if it were not for the tireless devotion they showed their dad he would not be here today. And to Nikki and Tony, we can only hope that their prayers were with their father when he needed them the most.

We are so very devoted to Mayo Clinic. Without question, extraordinary medical attention was always paid to Michael when it was essential. If not for their remarkable diagnosis of alpha-1 antitripsin deficiency and their excellent conscientiousness in the treatment of Michael's liver disease, the deadly pancreatic cancer that invaded his body would not have been found in a timely fashion. Their team of impressive specialists worked quickly and thoroughly to make sure the aggressive cancer that attacked my husband was eradicated. We are so very appreciative to Mayo Clinic, and to their amazing group of physicians who performed the surgery and prescribed the necessary protocol that was administered to prevent the return of the dreadful disease and ultimately save Michael's life.

We are immeasurably appreciative to Sarasota Memorial Hospital and their multitude of wonderful physicians and custodians. From their very efficient emergency room to their hospital wards; whenever needed, they took care of my husband in his darkest hours.

Michael and I are so very grateful to our donor and his family. It is difficult to express in words the feelings we have except to say that the gift of life they have given so unselfishly will always be cherished and held dear to us. We will forever pray for our donor and those he has left behind.

Last and most importantly, our deepest appreciation goes to Cleveland Clinic, whose humanitarianism and concern for the welfare and happiness of those who cross their threshold is essential in all facets of their health care programs. Was it timing, chance or luck that their team of professionals decided to accept Michael for a liver transplant? I don't think it was any of those elements. He is here today because of the judgment, compassion and wisdom of the many fine people on their staff who viewed him as an individual, not a number or statistic. My narrative is a tribute to the generosity of that great institution whose doctors and cast of participants gave my husband a chance at life when over 20 other hospitals would not accept him. We are indebted to the host of physicians whose technical expertise saved his life, to the many nurses and caregivers whose unwavering ministrations helped his recovery, to the experienced and proficient transplant staff who were and will always be there for us. The diligence and attentiveness that Cleveland Clinic's transplant program shows their patients is astounding. How can we ever thank them enough for saving Michael's life?

Our story of love, hope and survival is written for all of the above.

Time is too slow for those who wait,

Too swift for those who fear,

Too long for those who grieve,

Too short for those who rejoice,

But for those who love, *time is eternity.*

Henry van Dyke
(1852-1933)

Foreword

SECOND CHANCES

.

Everyone deserves a second chance. Second chances come about in many different ways and are always a precious gift. It could be a second chance at a career, a second chance to be a parent, a second chance for love or even a second chance at life. In medicine, second chances at life are really the most precious gift. Of course, we'd like to be able to say that it's within our power to give everyone a second chance. The sad fact of the matter, however, is that circumstances can oftentimes be cruel.

The first screening a potential transplant patient gets at a program is when the intake team screens a candidate's records. Unfortunately, at many centers there are trigger issues that exclude a candidate from further consideration and they are promptly rejected prior to any formal face-to-face evaluation. Michael Fayne had one of those trigger issues; he was a survivor of pancreatic cancer. His life's journey had taken him down a devastating path to where he and his family had just about exhausted all options and hope. But incredibly, they held on and continued to search for answers.

At Cleveland Clinic we recognize that each person's story and situation are unique and strive to minimize screening rejections. It is far better (but more labor intensive) to get the granular details of a patient's history and condition and make a deliberative and well-informed decision after a formal full evaluation at a multi-disciplinary candidate selection committee. These are rigorous and tough meetings; people's lives are on the line. Who gets the second chance? We have rules we have to go by, but it's never black and white. That's when we dig even deeper, get the real details and synthesize all the data into a probabilistic prediction of short and long-term success; looking to assure that with fairness and realism, we help patients and their families experience a second chance at life's journey together.

I believe that is what Susan and Michael experienced at Cleveland Clinic. They have asked me repeatedly why we saw things differently than over 20 other centers and gave him a chance. While I explained the process outlined above, we are also guided by an ethos of trying to err on the side of life and give people a second chance at life. That is the ethos that makes our team get up each day and be excited to go to work and what makes many of our patients friends for life. Three years later, I know I have two new great friends in Susan and Michael!

Charles Miller, MD

Director, Liver Transplantation

Cleveland Clinic

Possible Miracle

PROLOGUE
September 2012

I thought he had been dozing when Michael looked up at me from his hospital bed, asking in the weakest of childlike voices, "Am I going to die?" My heart was breaking as I held his face in my hands and lied, "No, no, no, you are going to be fine." When he finally drifted off to sleep my emotions could no longer be hidden while memories of the past came flooding back. My entire being ached for the man who had been the love of my life and the pillar of our family for more than 30 years. Thoughts of losing him crept into my mind along with images of living my life alone. It angered and terrified me all at the same time, but mostly it saddened me. I stared through a blur of tears at my husband's gaunt face and frail body picturing him as he had once been; so handsome and so strong both physically and mentally. Feeling pure anguish, I grieved for the happiness we once had shared together as I allowed myself to wallow in self-pity.

What was wrong with me? How could I not fight for Michael? He was deteriorating before my eyes while I looked on, helplessly hoping. Was I really that incapable? Was I really going to just let him die? My thinking was slowly evolving into soul-searching. It was at that moment I realized that living in the safe state of denial that had been my existence from the time my husband became ill was no longer a choice. I needed to be more than a good caregiver; I needed to be his advocate. I needed to find that tenacious, brave girl that lived inside of me. I needed to do whatever it took to save his life. Now more than ever I had to keep my faith and find hope. I prayed to God for the courage and strength I would surely require for what I was about to undertake. As I contemplated my insurmountable mission, determination surged through me in spite of the great trepidation and fear I was feeling. Even though I didn't know where to start, I knew in my heart there had to be someone, somewhere who could help Michael. Thus began my search for a *possible miracle.*

But the questions remained: How? Where? Who?

Chapter 1

A CHILD STAR
1943

I wasn't part of Michael's life when a dire genetic condition began working its evil on his tiny body. He was just a newborn when he first exhibited signs of an abnormality due to an unknown liver disease. The jaundice was unexplainable, as were the numerous other symptoms. When there wasn't a clear answer as to how the affliction was to be treated, his mother, upon the advice of his pediatricians, took her baby boy to see a well-known pediatric liver specialist in Boston.

World War II was still raging when Michael's mother made the arduous journey from Detroit to Boston by herself, on a train crowded with soldiers. She loved telling the story of how she held her infant for hours in her arms during the long ride. Once there, she stayed with distant relatives while her son was admitted to Boston Children's Hospital.

The pediatric gastroenterologist, likewise, did not understand why the otherwise healthy baby was showing signs of early liver disease. What the doctor did know was that Michael was in danger of losing his life. How absolutely terrifying this must have been for his mother when it was decided that exploratory surgery was the only course of action to try and save him. They operated on the infant's liver, not knowing whether he would live or die.

Michael never found out exactly what the surgery entailed and there was never a diagnosis as to the cause of his illness. Nevertheless, the procedure was a complete success, for he grew into a normal young man. The only reminder of his time in Boston was a significant scar he retained on his abdomen. No one understood until years later that the surgery was experimental, and therefore written about in the medical journals in 1943. I didn't know I married a "child star".

See hospital records on page 218 to view Michael's surgical and pathology reports from March 1943.

Chapter 2

SUSAN AND MICHAEL

1980 to 2000

At a very young age, Michael and his brother Ronnie were running a successful travel business. At 36 he had been married twice and, with his second wife, had two small children: Tony, 6, and Nikki, 4. He was a capable, controlling and handsome man with a charming, energetic personality that drew people to him. His zest for life was something to be admired. Being a self-made entrepreneur, he had few constraints, was able to do pretty much as he chose and certainly enjoyed that freedom.

When Michael and I first met, I was in the process of getting divorced from my first husband, whom I had married after living at home with my parents for 19 years. I was barely 20 and he was 24. After several years of marriage, we had grown apart. Suddenly I found myself a single mother. With eyes wide open, I felt no man would ever want to get involved with a 34-year-old woman who had three young children: Amy, 13, Adam, 9 and Darren, 7. I knew nothing of finances, didn't have a well-paying job, and had no plan of action. Living day to day, I had no idea what the future would hold for me and did not want to contemplate what my fate might be. People would ask me, "How will you manage?" My answer was always the same, "one day at a time." I remember vowing to never again let myself be found without control or direction in my life.

In 1980, while Michael was enjoying his freedom, I was scared to death of mine. The time of the flower child was coming to a close and self-awareness programs were flourishing. It was fitting that we were introduced during one of those meetings, as we were both searching: me to find myself, and he to find women.

The attraction was mutual and immediate when our paths first crossed, but we were both reluctant participants. He was a wild and cocky guy. I liked that about him. The song by Carly Simon "You're So Vain" was appropriate to describe his persona. As for myself, I was standoffish and aloof. He liked that about me. Because we had both lived with challenges in our past relationships, we tried to keep our distance. There was a mutual suspicion, so we did the dance that two divorced adults usually do: dating and trying to discover a reason to trust one another. On one of our initial dates, my new man told me, "There is no way I would ever marry again, especially a woman with three children." No surprise there: It was expected. In any case, marriage was off my radar, too. It was a slow push-and-pull process with my friends constantly reminding me I was wasting my time with lover boy. I didn't care because, when we were together, it was just plain old fun. We were becoming good friends, if nothing else. Eventually we brought our two families together and that was also fun. We were *The Brady Bunch* with all the same trials and tribulations.

During that period in my life, I was forced to move my children out of the house they had grown up in, as I couldn't afford the cost. I found a two-bedroom rental townhouse that suited us and set up our home. There was ample room for four plus a dog. It had two bedrooms on the upper level with an adjoining bathroom. The boys shared one room and Amy was in the other. I took over the small den on the first floor as my bedroom. The good news was that I was making a modest living, able to handle my own bills and proud of that accomplishment. Michael was very sweet during that time, for he knew that, although I needed it, I would not accept any money from him, either as a gift or as a loan. To compensate, he would come by from time to time bearing presents. He was our Santa. When he saw we didn't have a microwave, he bought us one. When he noticed our towels were in shreds, he showed up at our door with a mishmash of them in all styles and colors. He would take us out to dinner and on vacations with his children, making sure we were all comfortable and having a good time. He became my adviser in all things having to do with my finances and the kids' adviser in all things having to do with their social life and school. I, in turn, made him the family dinners that he craved. There was little else I could do to repay his generosity.

As time marched on, one year became two and two became three. In year four of our relationship we were kind of living together. Michael had a newly built home in the next suburb, but I had the kids, so he would spend the night with me on a regular basis, leaving early in the morning before they woke up. We thought we were hiding it from them. Of course, that wasn't the case and ultimately we came out of the closet and he moved in with us, giving up his house. With five of us, quarters became more cramped, especially for Michael who was used to his own space. There was little room for anything extra, so he was forced to keep his many suits in a portable wardrobe that collapsed like clockwork several times a week.

Being the controlling person that he was, he wanted to take over all of my expenses the day he moved in. I won't tell you that it wasn't tempting, because it really was. However, remembering the oath I had made to myself, I refused, allowing him only to pay for groceries, dry cleaning and other such things. He didn't like it, but it was the way it had to be for my self-esteem. I couldn't find myself worrying about money and floundering again.

The weekends that we had all the children together in my small town house were joyous times, although very chaotic. Tony would move in with Adam and Darren, while Nikki shared a room with Amy. They all had great attitudes, given the tight accommodations. The boys seemed to form a bond and Amy became sort of a mentor to Nikki, because she was like an older sister. Everything was very simple then.

After close to a year of "living in sin," Michael suggested that he buy a larger home that we all could live in more comfortably. It sounded good, but I told him I wouldn't leave the school district we were in, as I had made a promise to my children that they wouldn't have to change schools again the way they had to after my divorce. He agreed. I also explained that he would have to ask all the kids how they felt about his proposal. The five children had already paid a price with the many disruptions in their lives and that hadn't been fair to any of them. He agreed to that too. We were especially concerned about Nikki and Tony. They were babies when Michael got divorced and consequently had not lived with him for very long, so we knew it would be hard on them if Michael moved into a home that he owned, with my children, as it would seem more permanent; our town house arrangement had the appearance of being temporary. All the kids were older then and had opinions of their own. We would have to talk to all five. It's funny, when we were young we needed the blessing from our parents. At that juncture in our lives it was important to get the blessing from our kids. Only time would tell if we handled it well. The one thing I can say is that both of us loved our children unconditionally, and because of that love we did the best we could during that period.

Michael spoke with Tony and Nikki first to explain our plan, which included both of them having a place with us wherever we moved. He felt they were agreeable with that arrangement. Again, only time would tell, as they were still relatively young. Then at dinner one night he broached the subject of moving into a new home with my children, explaining that they wouldn't have to change schools again and everyone would have his or her own room. Adam and Darren were thrilled with the prospect of a larger house and a backyard. "Could we have a basketball hoop?" they asked. "No problem," he answered. Amy, however, had a different take on the topic. She, in turn, asked accusingly, "What if you decide you don't want us there one day? Or you don't like my mom anymore? What happens if you tell us to leave? Where would we go then?" The questions of my teenager revealed her pain and her fear. I felt it in my bones. "No," I told Michael later that night, "we will not be moving." So, we continued to live as we were for a while longer. All in all, our family was good then and I really didn't want anything else. I was in love and I knew Mickey (my affectionate name for Michael) was too.

As time went on, the familial situation worked itself out little by little. Then one day we were with all the kids on a vacation when out of the blue Nikki blurted out, "How should I introduce Susie to my new friends?" I cautiously told her, "I will always be your special friend." Not a great answer. That was it. One morning after we got home Michael woke up, looked at me and said, "It's time." "Time?" I asked. "I want us to be married. Call your mother. It's time everyone knew," he excitedly told me. I didn't think I could be happier than I had been, but I was. We prayed our children would adjust to the significant change that was about to occur in their lives.

We were going to have a small wedding but all the kids wanted a party, so we acquiesced and planned a real celebration. The invitation began:

> *Amy, Adam, Darren, Tony and Nikki invite you*
> *to the wedding of their parents Susan and Michael*

And so we were married October 6, 1985. We both cherished the very special relationship we had. I filled Michael's heart as he did mine. We really didn't need the piece of paper to know how committed we were to each other. There was no question of our love.

As he had promised, Michael bought a house in our current school district. Each of the kids had a section of the home that was theirs. Amy, who was off to college, had her own area in the lower level waiting for her whenever she returned. Darren and Tony were close in age and friends, so they shared a two-room suite. Adam had his own smaller room, as did Nikki. The family flourished in our new surroundings. Because Michael was my husband, I let him oversee all money matters. It was extremely easy for me to relinquish control and natural for him to take over.

Amy had the most difficulty with the new arrangement. From the beginning she made it clear that she didn't like Michael around. She felt that he was interfering in her life and taking me away from her. I tried to placate her with little success. Michael made a decision to handle the problem himself and he did. To this day I don't know exactly what he said to the young lady, but her attitude turned around afterward.

During that time Michael was becoming a calmer and more patient person. He was never at a loss when it came to giving advice to any of our children, whether they wanted it or not. He tried his best to be a good father and "stad" (my kids' name for him, short for step dad). Were things perfect? No, but we tried our best to make it close.

Michael's business continued to do well and I opened a ladies' boutique with my best girlfriend. When our lease was up, we closed our store. Michael dreamed of being in the restaurant/bar business. We eventually became partners in one tavern and then another. I took over owning the two taverns and managing a great number of employees, while Michael continued his work in the travel industry.

Sometime during our first few years of marriage, Michael decided to buy life insurance. A physical exam and routine tests were required before the application could be finalized. Upon getting the results of the blood tests the insurance agent called his office, asking my husband in a secretive voice if he was alone. After he secluded himself, the agent informed him that the insurance request had been denied due to his excessive drinking, inferring that my husband was an alcoholic. The blood analysis had shown unusually high liver enzymes. Michael assured the agent that alcohol wasn't an issue for him, although he did drink socially. It was agreed that he would take the test again in a few months and abstain from all alcoholic beverages in the meantime. After complying, the round of tests was repeated. Once again the liver enzymes were elevated. With a fair amount of concern Michael went to see his internist, who confirmed Michael had some cirrhosis of the liver, but that the cirrhosis had been present as long as he had been his doctor and that it was most probably leftover from when he was a baby. Several years before, the same physician had told him that he had to stop smoking, as he was developing emphysema. Our doctor didn't connect that revelation with the elevated liver enzymes and certainly not with the operation Michael had on his liver when he was an infant, so we all simply forgot about it.

We lived happily in our Michigan home for 14 years. The children became independent, went to college, got jobs and married wonderful partners, who together gave us eight phenomenal grandchildren. We had raised a terrific family, and felt it was our time now and we wanted to live it. Michael and Ronnie sold part of their business and we sold both restaurants. We changed our style of living, moving onto an old stately boat, *Eternity*, in Longboat Key, Florida. When we weren't there or visiting our kids, we were traveling the world: going on fantastic journeys to anywhere that you could imagine. It was surely a fairy tale existence.

We felt so very blessed that it was an easy decision to start helping others. Joining the National Disaster Team of the Red Cross was the perfect choice for us. After taking several necessary classes, we committed to work a month at a time when there were people that needed our assistance. We traveled the country from Alabama to Georgia to Louisiana to Ohio and more, giving aid. We saw first hand what it was like to lose everything, including loved ones, which made us all the more thankful for what we had. We learned to be giving individuals in a whole new way. It was the most rewarding, worthwhile undertaking I can ever remember experiencing. Working side by side and sharing that time with Michael made it all the more special.

We were intoxicated with life, spending all our time together, doing whatever we pleased. What could be better? What could go wrong? I remember being so very happy at that time of our lives, but I had an uneasy feeling that something could happen to change that.

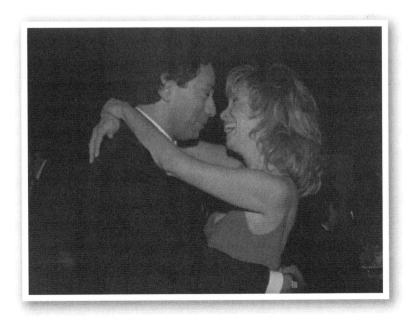

Chapter 3

WHAT IF? WHAT NOW?

2000 – April 2009

After selling his business Michael took a position with the large travel company that had purchased his. The new job entailed him working for the airline they owned, which was based in Minnesota. He commuted to Minneapolis from Longboat Key for a few days every week and I accompanied him on many of those trips. We hadn't established doctors in Florida where we lived, so it was simple for us to go to Mayo Clinic in Rochester, Minnesota, for routine physical exams. In early 2000, we entered their wellness program as a way to monitor our health.

It was at Mayo Clinic, when Michael was in his 50s, the doctors addressed the elevated liver enzymes. Specialists were called in and additional tests were ordered. We were both shocked when he was diagnosed with alpha-1 antitripsin deficiency, a genetic liver disease given to him by both his parents. That condition was the very root of his liver disorder when he was a baby. We learned it was also the cause of the cirrhosis and emphysema, as well as the reason for the elevated liver enzymes. The genetic malady was left unnamed until 1963 when it was discovered. Because Michael was feeling great and displaying no noticeable symptoms, he had been left undiagnosed. Through various scans the specialists found the cirrhosis of the liver was very prevalent and very likely increasing in his adult body.

As dictated by protocol, the physicians at Mayo started following the unusual and life-threatening affliction quite intently with a multitude of tests that were done annually. Michael was assigned to a gastroenterologist/hepatologist for his liver disease and a pulmonologist, as the cirrhosis of the liver adversely affects the lungs and he was at risk of developing COPD (chronic obstructive pulmonary disease). On his first visit, the pulmonary doctor told him, "Don't worry. If you have a problem with your lungs I'll get you a new set." I thought that sounded absurd and way over the top.

My paramount fear was losing my husband and the extraordinary life we had together. We initially became overcome with feelings of panic and dread. In time, however, we somehow learned to live with the diagnosis, as Michael didn't have any ill effects from the disease. Additionally, being watched so closely at Mayo Clinic, where the best doctors in the world were taking care of him, was comforting. Soon, any thoughts of complications from alpha-1 antitrypsin deficiency faded to the recesses of our minds as we went on living.

Before long… our nightmare began without warning. We were at Mayo Clinic in Rochester, where as per protocol for Michael's genetic affliction, an MRI of his liver was being performed. The tail of his pancreas, by pure coincidence, appeared in the corner of the image. The radiologists saw a small cyst that they suggested be investigated further. All the doctors thought it was benign, like most are, but they wanted him to have an endoscopic ultrasound strictly as a precaution. The procedure would entail the ultrasound to be done internally, through the esophagus under anesthesia. Michael didn't like the idea and he felt no urgency in having it done, so he wanted to go directly home. Even though I felt it was nothing to be concerned about, I wanted to stay at Mayo and get it over with. Of course, we did it his way, leaving for Florida without a resolution. I was extremely irritated and displeased.

We were home for a week when our gastroenterologist/hepatologist, Dr. Jack Gross, who by then was a good friend, called, persuading my stubborn husband to have the endoscopy done sooner rather than later. Even though he thought everything was fine, he reasoned a more definitive answer was in order. We chose not to question the slight change in his thinking. Because we were back home and didn't want to travel to Rochester for the test, the decision was made to have it done at Mayo Clinic in Jacksonville, Florida. I was glad I could stop nagging Michael about having the endoscopic ultrasound.

Within a short time the two of us were on our way to Jacksonville. Upon arriving we met the gastroenterologist/hepatologist who would be doing the procedure the next day. He felt, as the doctors in the North did, that the particular type of tiny cyst Michael had was benign. On Friday morning, without a care in the world, he was wheeled away to have the endoscopy while I spent my time reading, chatting on the phone and wondering where we would be having dinner that evening.

Awhile later the doctor appeared and summoned me into a smaller private anteroom. Without much ado he delivered a bombshell. During the endoscopy they had discovered the cyst on the pancreas to be a cancerous tumor. Feelings of pure horror engulfed me. "The doctors in Rochester had said it was nothing to worry about!" I managed to say, willing him to be wrong. However, they had not only done the ultrasound, but a biopsy of the tumor had been taken and tested, so there was no point in doubting the results. It was pancreatic cancer! To say I was astounded would be an understatement. I became numb;

I couldn't digest the information. I was terrified! My husband had pancreatic cancer, one of the worst forms of cancers known to mankind. Just the word cancer was more than I could bear let alone the pancreatic type. It sounded like a death sentence to me. I couldn't lose Michael! To make matters worse, my very best friend and confidant wasn't there to console me or help me through the horrendous turn of events. He was in a dreamland somewhere behind a myriad of curtains with thoughts of who knew what, although I can assure you, having cancer wasn't one of them. I was very much alone.

Just when my brain was starting to function again the doctor informed me he had to go. "Go?!" I repeated. Surely not before he told Michael the life threatening news. Oh yes, he had another procedure to do. To make matters worse, the nurses were not going to deliver the awful tidings to him, either. Then the doctor was gone and I was by myself thinking about how I was going to tell the man I loved that he had one of the most deadly forms of cancer. He would be absolutely scared to death. I remember sitting in that hideous little room alone, crying my eyes out and feeling so cold.

As soon as I gathered the courage I needed, I called our family. It took them time to take in the devastating diagnosis. In the meantime, Michael didn't have a clue about the cancer and there was no plan as to what we were going to do next. I told them that I would call back when I was able to assimilate all the information and knew how we were going to proceed.

I hated breaking the distressful revelation to Michael. I couldn't do it; I couldn't tell him. However, there was no choice. When he woke up asking me how the procedure went, I was the only one there to answer his question. I don't remember exactly what I said. I do know that I told him as gently as I could. Thankfully, he was still pretty groggy at the time. It wasn't until later in the day that we were both able to completely absorb the cancer diagnosis. Together we cried. Together we were so scared. Together we needed to make a plan.

There were so many questions. "What were we going to do?" was the first one. When the doctor had delivered the frightening pronouncement, he said that Michael needed surgery immediately. I had been catatonic and afraid at the time; not able to form my thoughts correctly. Once I had calmed down back at our hotel, I was ready to act. We were at Mayo Jacksonville, so it made sense to get in touch with the very same doctor who had done the endoscopic ultrasound earlier to see if the operation could be scheduled at their hospital as soon as possible, but it was late on a Friday and it took forever for him to call back. When he finally reached us, we were informed that the team that specialized in that kind of surgery was out of the country. "All of them at one time? You have got to be kidding me!" I argued, but he assured me that was the case. Of course, we had tried to reach Jack, Michael's gastroenterologist/hepatologist, who would surely know what to do, but he was unavailable too. So, we did as most people do in those situations: we played the "what if, what now" game over and over again, and then got the biggest pizza we could find.

Chapter 4

THE MIRACLE BOY

May 2009

There was no way the two of us were staying in Jacksonville over the weekend. We packed up and headed home where we spent an agonizing, sleepless weekend counting the minutes until Monday arrived. The time went so slowly, while unanswered questions did nothing but accumulate. The more we waited, the more foreboding and disbelief there was between us. Being too filled with fear to check out pancreatic cancer on the Internet, I chose to not address it. I'm not sure whether Michael did or not. All we could do together was go on and on, talking endlessly about all the ramifications of the disease.

Finally, Monday arrived and Jack called us back. When the shock of learning about the cancer wore off, he quickly went to work, first confirming the diagnosis with the Mayo Jacksonville doctor, then scheduling the surgery for that week in Rochester. The next morning we were on our way to Mayo Clinic.

The day after we arrived was spent doing blood tests, X-rays and various scans in preparation for the ominous event. When the testing was finished, we found ourselves sitting in front of a well-respected and accomplished surgeon, Dr. Florencia Que, whose specialty was pancreatic cancer surgery. She was pretty factual, wasting no time on bedside manner; we had Jack for that. After she went over the test results and examined Michael, she recited to us a litany of things that could go wrong. Among them was the scariest of scenarios: She would be looking for cancer in, on and around his other organs before the actual operation on the pancreas began. When she started, if she saw more lesions, the operation would be stopped and it would be all over in an hour. It would mean that Michael would not survive for very long because the cancer had spread. If everything went well it would last approximately three hours. The plan was to get rid of the tumor by taking off the distal end of the pancreas and collect several lymph nodes that would be later tested for cancer cells. It was way too much to absorb. Our tension was palpable as we left the office depressed and traumatized with more information than we had bargained for.

The crisis had the impression of occurring in a blur of double time. I couldn't catch up. Everything was taking place too fast. I was a walking, talking zombie, and Michael was in a state of shock. My sister Sally and brother-in-law Michael arrived at Mayo to be with us for the operation and for support afterwards. We spent a restless night holding each other, not believing what had happened to us in less than a week and trying like hell to be optimistic. Early the next morning we went to the hospital where my husband was admitted. All the while I willed myself to hold back my tears and hide my worry.

Our grandson had braided his papa a bracelet called a Wishlet the year before. When he tied it on his wrist, Michael made a wish. When the Wishlet gets so worn it falls off naturally, the wish is said to come true. As Michael was being checked into the hospital, he noticed that his Wishlet was missing. He freaked out because he couldn't remember his wish and took it as a bad omen.

We looked for it high and low but it was useless; we couldn't find it. I tried to convince him that he had surely made a good wish and it was a positive sign. He certainly had a lot to wish for in the hours to come.

We were taken to a small room where the preliminary preparations for surgery were done. With our emotions raw and before I was ready, Michael was telling me he loved me while being taken away. For his sake, I had been fighting for composure over the last week. When his gurney left the room it wasn't surprising that I lost it, and not in any small way. Watching him leave left me panic-stricken. He was so scared; who wouldn't be? I would have gladly taken his place. Being engulfed with thoughts of gloom and doom I sat in the pre-op room frozen, sobbing uncontrollably, until an understanding nurse took over, leading me to the surgical waiting area.

My husband was having major surgery: a pancreatectomy. I was under no delusion that the surgeon would also operate on or remove whatever else she deemed necessary. The wait was grueling. The nurse who had moved me into the surgical waiting room was getting updates from the OR on a regular basis. The operation was going fine, but the reports did little to abolish my misgivings. At first I didn't want to see the surgeon come out. It would mean the worst had happened and there was more cancer. After two hours I started to relax a bit, because I knew that she was going ahead with the surgical plan. After three hours the apprehension quickly came back. The torment heightened as every hour went by. The stress was palpable; I had never felt anything like it before. While my poor sis was knitting, I cried and carried on, and the more I cried and carried on the faster she knit. I remember saying over and over again, "Something is really wrong!" Watching families come and go after meeting with their surgeons caused the worry to escalate. My day was spent staring at the surgery board that indicated hour after hour the operation to be ongoing.

I had no patience. I wasn't prepared. I was a crazy woman. I expended most of the time bugging the nurses at their station. It was not my nature, but I did it anyway, sure that they were not telling me everything.

At long last, after six hours, it was over. The nurse who had been assigned to our case took me to a small private room, reminding me of the one in Jacksonville the week before and bringing back awful memories. The only thought I could entertain was that the surgery had gone badly and that was why it took so long. The negative feelings abounded as my whole body shook from the nervous tension. I couldn't even hold the glass of water I had been given. Waiting for the surgeon to arrive was almost as bad as waiting the six hours during the surgery. When she finally came into the room I looked at her face knowing immediately it had gone better than I was expecting.

I'm a good news, bad news kind of person, but I always want the bad news first, so I can have my happy ending. Even though Dr. Que had a smile when she first appeared, I knew that all wasn't rosy. With much more TLC than she had shown in our first encounter, she didn't disappoint. Starting with the bad news, she told me that Michael had the deadliest of cancers, as it was an extremely aggressive type. For that reason, his spleen had been removed as a precaution and was why the surgery had been unusually long. Continuing, she informed me that the prognosis for the type of cancer my husband had wasn't good; two years was the life expectancy. I felt as if I'd been stabbed in the heart. Then she added that if no cancer developed for the next five years, she felt he would have a good chance of surviving. I hated those goals. We rarely kept secrets from one another, but I chose to keep the revelation of that timetable to myself, as I knew Michael would never be able to handle it. How was I going to live with that kind of knowledge by myself? I really didn't know. There was also good news. The cancer wasn't in the head of the pancreas where the ducts are located. In fact, there was no sign of cancer anywhere else and she felt it had been caught in its earliest stage. I tried like hell to focus on the positive details of her report rather than the negative. Upon leaving the room she added, "Do not look up pancreatic cancer on the Web. Your husband's case is very much different than what you will find reported there. Pancreatic cancer is rarely found as early as his was. Michael is a very lucky man." With that she was out the door. Although I was tempted in the weeks to come, I took her advice and never looked it up.

More affirmative yet was Michael's recovery, which was amazing. Everyday when the doctors came to see him, they gave us encouraging information. The small tumor was encapsulated in the pancreas and the tail was cleanly removed, all 40 lymph nodes they had taken from his body tested negative for cancer cells and his spleen tested negative, confirming what Dr. Que had told me: Michael was a lucky guy. He was considered cancer free. The staff at Mayo Clinic called him a "'miracle boy". I tried to focus on that and not think about the time frame comments the surgeon had made to me.

Then one day just when I thought maybe we would be able to put the cancer behind us and go on with our life, an oncologist showed up at the miracle boy's bedside. I guess I didn't want to acknowledge that he may need additional treatment because everything was going so well. The protocol for pancreatic cancer, even after successful surgery, is a combination of chemo and radiation. However, we learned it was a preventative, elective measure, not necessarily life saving or mandatory. No one knew if he actually required it, for at the time there was no evidence of cancer. Nonetheless, because his type of cancer was the most aggressive kind and, if it were to recur, it would happen quickly, the doctor insisted Michael go through with the whole process, which would last about six months. In the beginning there would be chemo administered once a week for eight weeks, and then again at the end for another eight weeks. Halfway through the chemotherapy he would undergo six weeks of daily radiation and six weeks of continuous dosing of the chemo drug, night and day. I was curious as to how they would give him the chemo but didn't ask, as I already had enough information to absorb for the time being. The doctors were adamant that he have the middle part of the regime done at Mayo Clinic, as they had the very latest and best chemo and radiation equipment. The rest could be done in Sarasota with a local oncologist. All I wanted to do was shut the doctor up and make him stop talking. The whole process sounded horrendous and it took me awhile to assimilate the latest disturbing blow that had just been delivered. My hubby was still on drugs for pain, so I don't think he really grasped what the oncologist was adamantly recommending. Because he wouldn't start any of it for a month, Michael and I didn't talk about it then, which was perfectly acceptable as he was still recovering from the surgery.

After five days he was released from the hospital and shortly after that we left Rochester for home with Michael in a significantly weaker state. It was hard for us to believe all that we had been through in a matter of less than two weeks. By the time we got back on our boat, we were both shell-shocked.

In retrospect, it was a blessing in disguise that Michael had alpha-1 antitripsin deficiency and that Mayo Clinic had followed it so closely, or the cancerous tumor would have never been found. He would have surely died from the silent, deadly pancreatic cancer. Even after the horror we had been through, I felt blessed. I learned that it's not about having everything go perfectly all the time, but being able to face, with a bit of courage, that which goes wrong in life without losing hope. Together, we did that well.

Chapter 5

A HAPPY ENDING

June 2009 - June 2011

Once the surgery was over it was time for recuperation. I knew the docs wanted Michael in good shape before they attacked his body with chemo and radiation, so we spent our time doing exactly what they ordered: relaxing on our beautiful floating home, in our lovely marina, on our gorgeous island in the sun.

The convalescence was going quite well until one morning shortly after we got back. Upon waking, I heard my man cry out loudly. I tore down the hallway where I found him in the head (boat talk for bathroom) with a forlorn look on his face. As he glanced down I followed his gaze. We were both looking at Big Jim and The Twins who were black and blue with dark tinges of purple, oddly shaped and swollen to twice their normal size. His pride and joy was damaged beyond recognition. It was a sight to behold. If he weren't so unnerved by the incident, I would have had a good laugh. Immediately the panic button was pushed, with an emergency call made to Jack. Michael was more crazed about "the boys" than anything that he had gone through in the prior weeks. "It happens sometimes", Jack told my flipped out hubby. "The blood from the surgery drops down, pooling in the lower extremities." You think someone might have mentioned it beforehand, but I thought, "OK, I can deal with that kind of crap." However, I wasn't so sure Mickey could.

A month after the operation a scan of the surgery site was required to give the radiologists a baseline picture to use for comparison with future scans. Jack wanted it done at Mayo. Going north again didn't appeal to us, so we compromised, ending up back at Mayo Clinic in Florida. There we met with another oncologist who gave us another unwanted, unsettling eye-opener. Michael would need a port (central venous catheter) implanted in his chest for the chemo treatments. That type of permanent catheter placed into a vein was the best way to deliver the poison. When we went back to Mayo in Minnesota for the six weeks of chemo, the port was mandatory because he would be connected to a machine dispensing the drug 24 hours a day. I remembered after the surgery being told about that phase of the treatment, but I didn't realize the necessity of a catheter. I had thought he would have a simple IV. The recent turn of events rattled me. To put in the port, Michael would have to undergo another surgery. Although it was considered minor, I didn't like the thought of it at all. The doctor insisted we get the procedure done in Jacksonville as soon as possible. He assured us that it would be better for Michael to have the port for the many chemo infusions in the hard months ahead. There was no other reasonable option; the oncologist had made perfect sense.

Once again the whole conversation that day seemed to go right over Michael's head. I knew he had no memory of talking to the oncologist after his surgery regarding the treatment he would ultimately need. When we left the appointment I expected him to be upset about having to go to Rochester for six weeks of radiation and being connected to a chemo machine the whole time. The notion of it should have bothered him. It did bother me, but he didn't mention it afterward. Maybe with all that had transpired, it was too much for him to handle, choosing instead to block it all out of his mind. That was fine with me because at that point he didn't need his world rocked again.

Subsequently, I found myself in another waiting room while the catheter was being surgically inserted into a vein in his chest. It made what we were about to go through undeniable. A while later when we were in the recovery area together, I noticed another couple across the room. The man apparently had his port removed that day. They were celebrating the occasion and looked overjoyed to have his therapy over. When would that happy couple be us? We were clearly a long way from that time and definitely a long way from being happy.

While we were at Mayo Clinic in Jacksonville, the oncologist recommended a very accomplished oncologist in Sarasota, Dr. Caryn Silver. That's where we started the terrible chemo process. The poisonous chemical was administered through the catheter in Michael's chest into his body every week at her office. Blood tests and scans were done frequently, overseen by Dr. Silver and then sent on to Mayo Clinic for more scrutiny, where several doctors there checked the results of the scans and blood work. It was a non-stop search for cancer.

Our acute anxiety would start before the tests began and would last until we got the call that all was well from both our local doc and the Rochester doc. During the time in between, we would look at each other, knowing what the other was thinking: "What if they find something?" In the back of my mind was the timetable the surgeon had recited to me: The two-year cancer free goal that I had kept a secret.

Every scan was traumatizing, as were the many blood draws. One blood test was specifically for a pancreatic cancer marker called CA 19-9. If it rose it would mean that the cancer was active. As I mentioned previously, when the blood was drawn a portion of it was overnighted to the Mayo Clinic lab. The number in Sarasota was never the same as the one done in Rochester, even though it was from the very same blood sample. We were fixated on the outcome of that test. The fact that it was different and inconsistent made us freak out every time we got the results. Caryn and her assistant helped us manage through those profoundly difficult times. Michael did astonishingly well with only minor complaints during that period.

In the middle of the chemotherapy we went back to Mayo in Rochester for the abhorrent six-week stint, settling in a residential hotel. I knew it was not going to be fun for me, but when I thought of what Michael would have to endure, I felt sick. The testing and scanning started first to make sure all was satisfactory to go forward with the radiation and chemo as planned. Then we met with the radiologist and oncologist for tutelage on exactly what lay ahead. Both of us were oblivious to what we were about to live through in the next couple of miserable days.

The alarm was set off when the radiologist's physician's assistant came in to talk to us. It was evident by his demeanor that there was big trouble. He wasted no time informing us that a mass had been seen in the abdominal cavity on the pictures from the latest scan and that it was questionable as to the origin. My heart dropped, my head spun, my stomach lurched. I knew he thought that the cancer had come back.

We were both emotionally overwrought as we grasped the implication of the latest development. The doctors wanted to do an endoscopic ultrasound to see what it was. He confirmed what I had been thinking: The cancer may have come back. I remember the screaming in my head, "NO! NOT AGAIN!" There was no time for hysterics. Immediately Michael was sent to see the oncologist to verify the correct protocols to follow. He agreed with the radiologist. We were both dazed, but Michael was able to ask a question anyway. "What happens if they find more cancer?" I wanted to put my hands over my ears. I didn't want to know the answer. The doctor told us in a concerned sympathetic tone that if the mass turned out to be malignant there would be no radiation and no surgery, only chemo until Michael couldn't take it anymore. We both knew what that would signify. The oncologist confirmed our deepest fears. Michael wouldn't have a great deal of time left. We needed to be there for each other now more than ever. I tried like hell to hold it together.

It was a déjà vu experience for us. The endoscopic ultrasound was how the pancreatic cancer was diagnosed in the beginning of our ordeal. The very next day I kissed Michael as he was wheeled away for the same kind of ultrasound he had undergone a few months prior. The whole time I was remembering the two-year deadline and thinking the cancer had come back. It was another excruciating wait. The doctor who did the procedure came to talk to me as soon as it was over, but was non-committal about what he had observed. We would have to patiently bide our time for the lab results to be completed and the radiologists to look at the pictures that had been taken before a conclusion could be reached. Because it was a Thursday, there was a possibility we would not know anything until Monday. The oncologist couldn't have been more empathetic. Knowing how tortuous the anticipation was, he said he would push for the results as quickly as possible.

With Thursday gone, we were hopeful that we would hear the outcome of the endoscopic ultrasound the next day even though we knew it would be iffy. On Friday, with phone in hand, we wandered the city like robots, walking and waiting, and waiting and walking. Both of us had a despondent feeling regarding the test results, so much so that we couldn't even console each other. Standing on a street corner in the middle of the afternoon, the phone rang. Michael answered it immediately: The call was from his oncologist. The doctor asked him if he was sitting down, which my hubby took to mean the worst kind of news. Michael went down on his knees in the middle of the sidewalk. I followed his lead, thinking the same thought. However, it wasn't bad news at all. The ultrasound showed the mass to be scar tissue; a residual effect from the surgery. We went from depressed to ecstatic in minutes, as a rush of emotions paralyzed us. The nutty, jubilant couple sitting on a street corner must have been quite a sight for any passersby.

As insane as it sounds, we couldn't wait for the treatments to start. Who would have thought that instead of moaning and groaning about the impending chemotherapy and radiation, we were embracing it? We were happy and ended up having a festive night.

Since they were going ahead with the radiation, Michael had to have tattoos placed at the points on his torso where it would be administered. Once that was done, he was ready for his body to be blasted by radiotherapy. Every morning he went to the radiology department where he would lie on a table while their monstrous machine attacked his cells. At the same time, the gizmo that dispensed the chemo was hooked to the port in his chest. The toxic cocktail was pumped into his feeble body 24 hours a day nonstop, even while he slept. In the quiet of the night I could hear it humming as it attacked my husband. Once a week he would go to the clinic where the horrid thing was refueled and his labs were done. He wore the contraption in a fanny pack around his waist. It was difficult for someone as vain as Michael to handle and so hard for me to look at. All in all, he was a great patient with few grievances. The only side effect was weight loss. He was never nauseous nor did he lose much hair. My heart hurt for him the entire time he was enduring the torture at Mayo.

It seemed eons before the six weeks of misery were eventually over. There was little to be elated about during that period, but having the fanny pack with its atrocious machine removed made us both smile. At the same time the radiation phase was completed. There was a large bell in the clinic waiting room. When the radiation therapy for a patient was over they would ring the bell signaling the end of treatment. It caused camaraderie, as most of the patients in the room were there for the same reason: cancer. When the bell sounded, everyone clapped and cheered for the fortunate guy or gal who had completed their round of radiation. When it was Michael's turn, my man stood at the front of the room ringing the bell and crying like a baby.

When that agonizing stage of the hopefully lifesaving protocol was over, it was time to go home. Next on Michael's agenda was the continuation of the endless scans and blood tests, as the final part of the chemotherapy was completed. Once again it was done at our local oncologist's office with results from the labs and the scans sent to Mayo Clinic as the doctors continued their endless search for the return of the detestable pancreatic cancer. Living with stress had become part of our lives. All the angst was hard to take that first year.

At that time the doctors felt Michael should go for genetic testing. Even though his cancer wasn't linked to the alpha-1 antitripsin deficiency, we were surprised to learn that breast and pancreatic cancer are linked. There was a history of breast cancer on his father's side of the family causing some suspicion. Upon completion of the genetic testing we learned that Michael did test positive for a mutation in the BRCA2 gene, which in turn was the cause of the pancreatic cancer. It really didn't help him to have the information at that point in his life, other than to be vigilant about the possibility of getting breast cancer. More importantly, we both felt that it was essential for his children and siblings to know.

Upon meeting with Caryn after the final chemo treatment, she told us Michael had remained cancer free and there was no longer a need for the hated port. The day it was taken out was a monumental occasion. We had overwhelming feelings of happiness and freedom. The six months of torment were finally over. With a smile on my face I waited patiently while the port was being removed. When I went into recovery afterward and kissed my man, I thought of the other couple I had seen so many months ago celebrating. At that moment it was our turn.

Michael had remained emotionally strong through all those stress-ridden months. I was the one who fell apart. The mere mention of the cancer, surgery, radiation or chemotherapy sent me into a tailspin. The dilemma was that he needed to talk about it and I couldn't bear to hear anything regarding it. Listening to Michael reveal what he had been through to anyone and everyone had become intolerable for me. Caryn could feel and see how emotionally shaken up I was and recommended a therapist who specialized in PTSD (post traumatic stress disorder). I didn't think her diagnosis was correct and was sure that in time I would be fine. However, I went to see the psychologist anyway. She explained to me that I had been under extreme strain for hours during the surgery, as well as before and afterward. With her I had to relive every moment of that terrible time in our life. Eventually Michael joined me for the appointments, and when he saw my devastation when anything to do with his cancer was talked about, he became more sensitive and stopped referring to it as often. As an aid, she suggested that when I felt myself slipping and heading down that dark road, to picture a stop sign ahead of me and turn right or left to avoid going there. I have continued to use that tool. The therapist, along with Michael, helped me get over the most debilitating crisis in my life.

With the support of our wonderful family, friends and doctors we had both survived. Gradually Michael got over the effects of the chemo and radiation. Cancer was still a concern, but in time the tests and scans became fewer and further apart, as no sign of the disease was ever found.

Over the months and years that passed, thoughts of illness and dying slowly faded away. With our new lease on life we truly lived it. Our days couldn't have been more glorious. We started believing the cancer wasn't going to show itself again. The only thought of the surgeon's timeline was when there was an anniversary of the surgery. Slowly we made our way back to our usual lifestyle, living on our boat and traveling the world. Did I have my happy ending? I thought maybe I did.

Chapter 6

THE BEGINNING OF THE END

July 2011

In July 2011 we went to Mayo Clinic in Rochester for our annual physical exams. We had been concentrating on cancer and sort of forgot about the liver issue, which had a different set of diagnostic analyses required. Upon completing the appointments and needed testing, it is the process at the Clinic to meet with the primary physician for a review. For Michael, it was our pal, Jack, who reported that there was no sign of pancreatic cancer, which was always a relief. However, the MRI of the liver was not quite so definitive. The imaging had shown a minute spot on his liver. It had been seen before on prior pictures, but all of a sudden it was slightly larger than it had been previously. We hadn't been told about it, as no one thought it to be worthy of discussing. Neither Jack, nor the radiologists felt there was a need for concern. It was reminiscent of the pancreatic cancer discovery two years earlier. That supposedly was nothing to worry about either. The whole conversation gave me the chills.

Considering that Michael's liver function had remained stable throughout the past year and the fact that it was just a speck that was seen on the scan, Jack's recommendation was to continue watching the small spot in the months to come. To say I was uncomfortable with the new disclosure would have been an understatement. It was eerie how similar it was to the small lesion that was discovered on the pancreas. Since the doctors were not going to check it again for a while, we went home accompanied by a disturbing feeling.

I chose not to mention the latest development to any of our family. It is important to address the mystery as to why I didn't share information about Michael or ask our children to be with me for the multitude of unnerving events we had been through. It is a conundrum that I'm sure a therapist would have fun with. When I look back, there is no question that I desperately needed them with me and that they would have been there had I told them. If I had to guess, I would say that I thought that if I didn't admit to anyone, especially our family, that something was amiss, I wouldn't have to admit it to myself. Instead I wanted to think I was protecting them, but the real story was that I knew I could handle the situation better emotionally if I totally denied what was happening. Intentionally forgetting that they had every right to know about the health of their dad, I kept the truth from them. I hope they are able to forgive me for being so terribly selfish at that juncture in my life. We all have regrets and that is a big one for me. I have since come to want and need all the support and help they can give. I've realized how important it is to be able to share the bad times along with the good, not only with my husband, but also with our children.

Then Jack called. In the flash of a second our life changed, just as it had in the past with the cancer diagnosis. He had been at a conference where he shared Michael's case file with other gastroenterologist/hepatologists. There was agreement among the other specialists that the conservative approach should not be taken with the spot on the liver. It needed to be dealt with immediately. Although it wasn't said aloud, I wondered if he was thinking it could be liver cancer after all we had been through. I refused to believe it and we didn't ask.

In a few days we were back at Mayo Clinic sitting in Jack's office while he informed us that Michael was scheduled to undergo a minimally invasive procedure called an ablation. A radiologist would go into his liver with a long needle while following the process by CAT scan and simply burn the spot away with a laser. No cutting, no biopsy and no real answer as to what it was. Once again I was incredulous, numb and totally dazed.

Early the next morning we went to the same hospital where Michael had the pancreatic surgery. It was definitely bizarre for me to be back there and I know it was more so for him. Once we got to the check-in area, we found we had forgotten our insurance cards. I left Michael at the hospital and went to the hotel to retrieve them. On the way back, I ran into Jack. Standing there in the middle of the throngs of people outside the hospital entrance, I eagerly received his much-needed hug. He seemed to sense how anxious I was. Even though we were far from alone, without thinking, I blurted out a question I hadn't planned on asking, but one that must have been lurking in the recesses of my mind: "Is this the beginning of the end, Jack?" I wanted the reassurance he had always given me. I needed to know everything was going to be all right. I was terribly distressed by the unexpected liver complication. Jack had always been very positive about Michael's well-being and that's what I expected at that time. However, he never answered me, just hugged me even tighter than before, told me he would visit Michael in the hospital and then went on his way. His silence was deafening. A voice inside me said that it was a turning point. I knew that his non-answer had an implication of what was to come and that it wasn't good. Departing in tears I went to find Michael, trying not to think. The new revelation was filed away with the other undisclosed information that I had accumulated regarding my husband's health, information that I once again kept from everyone.

Back at the hospital I kissed Michael while the attendant took him away from me to have his body invaded anew. I walked the halls biding my time and blocking out the doubt-filled future. When it was over, the radiologist told me the ablation had gone perfectly; the spot was gone. He added that he couldn't determine exactly what it was. In a way I was glad. I didn't want to know. It felt so much better being oblivious.

A few days later Jack told us the consensus of opinion was that the small tumor had looked highly suspicious, as in cancerous, but not the pancreatic kind. That was semi-positive, although I had a feeling it was his way of not scaring the crap out of us. It was undeniable that all of a sudden the unwanted spot was now definitely being called a cancerous tumor. The casual change in wording caused my chest to tighten. He added that these small tumors were symptomatic of liver disease and that more of them may develop. Did he mean more cancer? I was traumatized! He continued that we shouldn't worry about it too much, because they could always be zapped away when they were discovered. Don't worry about something that was very likely liver cancer: an extremely difficult assignment. It was hard to hide the depression I was feeling. In any case, Michael recovered quickly, seemingly not to be as focused on the cancer issue as I was. My unanswered question to Jack caused me the most concern. I could not get it out of my mind. Was it the beginning of the end?

Chapter 7
DENIAL
September 2011 – March 2012

*M*ayo Clinic was seeing far too much of us. If I found the trips physically and emotionally exhausting, can you imagine how hard it was on my guy? It took him some time to recover from the last trek. When home again we tried to resume our routines along with our laid back life. The first thought was that we needed R and R, especially Mickey. Sally and Michael own a condo overlooking the Gulf of Mexico on Anna Maria Island in Florida. It's close to where we live and wasn't being rented at the time. A couple of weeks on the beach would surely make things better, but it didn't go quite the way I had hoped. We did go to the condo, but it was far from relaxing.

I have a hard time remembering when things started changing because it happened so slowly. Now, thinking back, I'm vague about when Michael really began spiraling downhill. The onset of the annoying, not life-threatening, symptoms appeared one at time. First, he began feeling unusually cold. In the heat of the Florida weather he would shiver and wear a sweatshirt. Then, the lethargy ensued. He would sit around all day doing nothing and then take a nap. That wasn't like him at all. Sometimes he felt feverish and achy, as if he was coming down with the flu. He also developed unusual itching, which became one of his worst symptoms. Much later we found out that it was called the "bilirubin itch," also caused by cirrhosis of the liver, but at that time we thought it was just dry skin. In addition, his urine appeared darker than normal. All the issues were due to his liver disease, although we didn't realize it then. Individually these phenomena didn't seem to be a sign of anything terrible and it was easy to reason them away as I kept inventing one plausible explanation after another. We tried to continue our life thinking everything would eventually be good again even though we had evidence to the contrary.

Then, the weight gain started at an incredible rate in a very short time. Was he eating too much? Was he was just getting fat? His belly was out of control. I pleaded, cajoled and begged him to do something about it. Finally, he started watching what he ate, but there was no change. In fact, he got even bigger, eventually not being able to button his pants.

The question as to why it was happening was answered before we were ready. Michael was taking his usual afternoon nap, and I was having a lazy day reading while waiting for him to get up. All of a sudden I heard him yell, "SUSAN" at the top of his lungs as he came running into the living room. It more than startled me. As he stood before me he dropped his shorts. Oh no, not those guys again! Yes, it was Big Jim and The Twins. I was speechless as it was not hard to see that they were misshapen and, once again twice the normal size and totally unrecognizable. What the hell had happened to those boys now? I calmed him down as he placed what was becoming a routine panic call about his pals. Jack concluded, after listening to Michael's tirade, that he had developed ascites. He explained that it was another symptom of liver disease caused by the cirrhosis. The liver wasn't functioning properly, thus the peritoneal cavity in the abdomen was filling with fluid. It is not uncommon for the liquid to collect in the belly and also in the legs, thus the weight gain. When I looked at Michael's calves and ankles, sure enough, I noticed that they were swollen. And, unfortunately for my poor honey, the fluid had found another place to accumulate.

That explained the potbelly, the weight gain and the odd shape of Big Jim and The Twins. Again, it was all about his liver, but the water retention was considered potentially serious. I was becoming so numb about what was going on that when Jack sent us to the ER immediately, I was not alarmed in the least. I was on autopilot. At Sarasota Memorial Hospital the diagnosis of ascites was confirmed. Blood tests were done to make sure the abdominal fluid was not infected. Luckily that wasn't the case. Liver damage can also cause low albumin levels. Albumin helps to keep fluid in the blood vessels and low levels can add to the excess liquid, so that was checked too. After a thorough exam, we were sent on our way with a prescription for a diuretic and told to come back if a fever developed. I couldn't believe that there was another problem to deal with and a potentially dangerous one at that, but I somehow managed to take it in stride.

The new ailment was not good. However, because the water pills did their job, we tried not to focus on it. In no time Big Jim and The Twins were back to normal, the tummy was going down and the ascites was being controlled. I thought the fix was going to take care of everything.

Then unexpectedly Michael was experiencing weight loss. We didn't anticipate that. It seemed maybe the diuretics were doing too much. His muscle mass was leaving him at a startling rate and he was becoming very weak. He couldn't work out like he had been doing just a month before. I got him

Ensure nutritional shakes and drinks and made all his favorite meals. Jack kept adjusting his meds trying to find the right cocktail. It seemed a fine line we were walking. Soon his health was in check as we learned to put a Band-Aid on every new problem that developed.

When we spoke with Jack, he confirmed that all the symptoms Michael was experiencing were not unusual for someone with alpha-1 antitripsin deficiency. Knowing that made it harder for me to just explain them all away. Surprisingly, both the liver function tests and the meld score, which is how the progression of liver disease is tracked, were at the high end of normal, even after the ablation. It gave us an unreasonable belief that the liver problems were seemingly resolved.

At the time I didn't understand or want to know what the meld score actually meant. I didn't grasp how incredibly significant it was in determining the advancement of liver disease. Nor did I realize that soon it would be an all-consuming number for me. I never researched any of it. We continued on with our life ignoring the warning signs. After all, Michael seemed to have beaten a dangerous cancer. Why couldn't he do the same with the liver trouble?

Because of these new turn of events we found it necessary to find a gastroenterologist/hepatologist in Florida. It was becoming hard for Jack to handle a potentially problematic illness long distance. We discovered a great physician, Dr. Isaac Kalvaria, who started routine exams, blood tests and, most importantly, was affiliated with Sarasota Memorial Hospital. I felt we were in good shape. Aside from some oral surgery he needed, Michael remained stable for several months. The ascites was under control as were the other signs of liver disease, so we started making travel plans.

Chapter 8

BLINDLY OPTIMISTIC
April 2012 – May 2012

From September 2011 to April 2012 Michael seemed to feel good, or at least as good as he could feel at that time. We did some traveling, hung out at home and he had some dental implant work done. Soon it was the end of April and we were heading to Michigan for our grandson's bar mitzvah.

We went north three weeks early so we could spend the Passover holiday with our family. Everything was going great, until without much warning, Michael's feverish symptoms that had been occurring from time to time turned into a full blown fever. Because of the nausea and lack of appetite he was experiencing, I assumed it was the flu. The more he stayed in bed the more worried I became and eventually started thinking that something else was going on. Contacting Jack seemed to be the way to go, as we didn't have a doctor in Michigan. After calling his office I learned that he was in Italy. It was hard finding a time to talk with him being overseas, so instead I texted him the pertinent information regarding Michael's status. Jack, being mindful that the ascites fluid could become infected, put him on an antibiotic. As luck would have it I carried the prescription with me just in case it would be needed. Michael started taking it immediately, but the fever persisted.

On the day of our grandson's service his health was still failing, with the fever even higher than it had been. He showed no signs of getting better. If anything, he was worse, barely being able to get out of bed or eat. After a flurry of texting, Jack wrote, "Take him to Mayo Clinic ASAP." Jack is not an alarmist, so I knew he thought Michael was in trouble. It was a scary time.

We missed the bar mitzvah. Disappointments happen in life, but that was a monstrous one. I was inconsolable and wanted to curl up into a ball. Of course, that wasn't even close to an option, because my husband needed me. Even though the rabbi arranged for us to watch the service via closed circuit TV, it did little to relieve the heartache I felt. My concern was so focused on Michael that I spent the rest of the night watching over him.

Early the next morning we flew to Rochester and went directly to the emergency room at Mayo Clinic, where Jack had arranged for a series of tests, including having the fluid in Michael's belly tapped. A long needle was used to go into the peritoneal cavity and draw out some of the liquid that had accumulated there. It was then checked for infection. All the tests came back negative. I was relieved that it didn't seem to be Michael's liver causing his illness. But what was going on? By then Jack was back from Italy. He scheduled a bevy of appointments with various medical specialists. None of the doctors could determine the source of the fever, which was peculiar considering Mayo Clinic is known for diagnostic capabilities. It was a real mystery. The infectious disease physician was the last of the appointments. He took a number of blood tests with all the results coming back normal. Just when we thought that all the possibilities had been exhausted, an idea came to mind. Could the fever have anything to do with the dental implants? The doctors thought it was worth looking into. Michael was sent to see an oral surgeon, who took some very sophisticated X-rays. The pictures showed the site of the implant to be infected and thus the cause of the fever. What a relief!

After being at Mayo Clinic for more than a week Michael was released to go home. He saw his local oral surgeon, who removed the implant. The change in him was incredibly fast. With the fever completely gone, he appeared to be good. He was still cold, tired and itchy, but he was tolerating it. The diuretics were controlling the ascites and although his energy level was not great, it was endurable. I thought he was really doing well, or at least that's what I chose to believe. Remission isn't a word used for liver disease. However, I was irrationally hopeful, as he was so much better than he'd been in weeks.

All his physicians gave us the thumbs up, so there seemed to be no reason we couldn't go on the cruise we had been planning. A few weeks later Michael and I were traveling and celebrating life again. We drove across the state to Ft. Lauderdale where we stayed in our favorite waterfront hotel. The days were spent going for walks and being lazy by the pool. Before the departure day we strolled down to the marina to look at the beautiful view. The apprehension of leaving the country was something we shared, given Michael's recent health concerns. As we stared out at the water we decided to call Jack for some reassurance. Without hesitation he gave us encouraging words, making us feel so much better about our voyage. He affirmed that there was no reason we shouldn't go. That was all we needed to hear to boost our confidence.

Soon we were cruising out of Ft. Lauderdale, crossing the Atlantic and starting our exciting journey from one fabulous, historic city to the next. It was wonderful exploring those old capitals of Europe together while enjoying the ship. However, the fun was short lived. Michael unfortunately developed symptoms

10 days into the trip. The change in him was slow and almost undetectable as he started becoming ill.

There was a friend of mine on the ship from previous travels. One day she asked me about the appearance of Michael's skin, commenting, "His coloring doesn't look right." What was she talking about? "That's how he tans!" I explained, overlooking the fact he now had a yellow tinge to his face, body and even the whites of his eyes. Then the itching he had been bothered with became insufferable, so much so that his skin was raw all over from scratching. It was probably from the cold weather, I convinced myself. We bought different types of moisturizers to combat the dryness. Speaking of cold weather, he became increasingly more chilled all the time. Wearing warmer clothes and turning the heat up temporarily took care of the problem. His fatigue also got worse, so nap time increased. The very most worrisome was the ascites. It started coming back, even with the diuretics, causing him to have difficulty breathing and eating, as the built up fluid pressed on his lungs and other organs. OK, still nothing we couldn't deal with; he was going to be fine.

I was trying to help get Michael's various disturbing issues under control when he developed a fever again and not just a low grade one. It was major, shakes and all. The high fever was much more severe than the previous one. We went immediately to the ship's hospital where he got great care from an experienced doctor and staff. After I explained his current liver problems, they drew blood to check for infection. I was texting Jack the whole time regarding Michael's condition. I sent him pictures of his belly that I took on my cellphone so he could assess the fluid buildup. At the same time, the ship's doctor faxed Jack the results of the blood work. It was amazing; we were halfway around the world and Michael was being monitored by Mayo Clinic. We spent the night in the ship's hospital, he was put on IV antibiotics and Jack had the dose of the diuretics increased. We knew it wasn't the oral surgery. Maybe the fluid was, in fact, infected, but they couldn't tap it on the ship because of the risk of an infection. I was relieved when in a few days he was much better. We never did find out the cause of the fever and I really didn't want to know.

Looking back, I ask myself if Jack told us to go on our vacation because he knew it could be our last one ever, that our chances of traveling together again were non existent. The thought occurred to me many times over the months to come. I started to think the fever Michael had in Michigan wasn't from the dental implant after all, that maybe there was more to it, and it was related to the fever on the ship.

The trip had become a disaster. From that time forward Michael was never himself and I mean never. The fever was gone, but the lethargy, sensitivity to cold and itching were steadily increasing, and the ascites was getting more severe. All were a constant irritant to my poor husband. We had to end our trip early, flying from Amsterdam to Atlanta before we went on to Sarasota the following day. Can you believe, after all that had happened, I was still convinced that Michael was going to be fine? It was insane to be a Pollyanna with all the warning signs, but that's who I was then. How could I continue to be so blindly optimistic about his decline?

Chapter 9

THE SLIPPERY SLOPE

Early June 2012

Upon arriving at the Hartsfield-Jackson Atlanta International Airport all I wanted to do was get to our hotel as quickly as possible. We were both in need of some down time, so we planned to spend the night there before flying home the next morning. Being seasoned travelers, we know how to navigate an airport. After deplaning, I quickly started walking toward the mass of people at Atlanta airport's immigration and customs. Shortly, I turned to say something to my partner only to find him missing. Searching the area I saw him, a long way off, lackadaisically strolling in my direction. I wanted to get out of the airport fast, but he obviously didn't have the same urgency. I don't mind telling you I was extremely irritated, which isn't my nature. I regrouped, went to him and asked what the problem was. He laughed and asked if there was some place he could sit down. It seemed we were having some miscommunication. In any event, we ended up in the back of a very long line with Michael not talking until he reached the immigration officer. There he started joking with a man who was in no mood for his nonsense. I couldn't believe the strange shift in his attitude and demeanor. I understand now that's when I was first introduced to the very worst symptom of his liver disease. Denial had become my new modus operandi, so I let it go as jet lag. It seemed a perfectly reasonable explanation.

When we finally got to the hotel my guy went directly to bed instead of having dinner with me as we had intended. I was dumbfounded because he had been out cold for most of the plane ride and hadn't eaten much, but glad he would be sleeping off the bout of malaise he seemed to be having. The next day we had an uneventful trip back to Florida.

Even though Michael seemed somewhat better once we got home, I remained unsettled by his behavior from the night before, my instincts telling me something new was at work on him and it involved his cognizance. Everything he did and said was slightly peculiar and not like him at all. I decided, on my own, to call my go-to doctor. Jack told me that he thought Michael was displaying early signs of hepatic encephalopathy. "Encepha . . . what in the world is that?" I asked dubiously, not wanting to consider there was yet another issue to deal with.

Apparently, the ammonia in his body wasn't detoxifying in his liver as it should because of the cirrhosis. The buildup of the toxins is typified by deterioration of brain function. So, Jack simply explained, the ammonia was going into his brain giving him the appearance of having had too much to drink. As my gut instinct had indicated, I was being introduced to yet another new sign of liver disease. Jack assured me the new phenomenon could be treated when it was time. It sounded threatening to me. "Just pile it on," I thought. I told Jack that the ascites was more evident than ever. He felt the meds needed to be adjusted once again, as the water pills were not working as they should. In the meantime, Michael remained unaware of my conversation with Jack or that there was another potential problem on the horizon. I knew he wouldn't take it well, so I chose not to address it with him until I thought he could handle it better. At that point I realized I was starting to take over my husband's care.

As soon as we were settled at home, we went to Isaac Kalvaria's office. Michael seemed good at the appointment. There was no outward sign of encephalopathy and no staggering around. He appeared normal to everyone but me, nevertheless I knew him better than anyone and could tell something wasn't quite right. I explained to the doctor what I had observed about my husband's manner and what Jack thought it might be. Mentioning the subject in front of Michael was clearly a mistake; my spouse wouldn't admit to feeling anything except fine and was exceedingly annoyed that I had talked about his actions. Was it possible Jack had been wrong about the ammonia accumulation? He was right about the water pills. They needed to be readjusted to control the fluid accumulation. After a thorough physical examination and checking his blood work, Isaac made a chilling comment to Michael, "You are on a very slippery slope, my friend!" I didn't know what he meant, but it sure made me shiver. I filed it away with thoughts of my unanswered "beginning of the end" question to Jack.

Isaac conferred with Jack after the exam. They both agreed that Michael should go to Mayo Clinic sooner rather than later for a complete work up. There were new questions regarding his health that needed to be addressed. I didn't ask what they were; I would find out soon enough. We had appointments scheduled for our physicals in a month anyway. With Jack's help it was all arranged. We were going back to Rochester again.

We had done the same drill a million times since we had become patients of the Clinic. A long day lay ahead of us. Driving to Tampa and staying in a hotel the night before always helped us make it through the exhausting trip, so that was what we did. The day we flew north we were up early and made our plane with little hassle. That all changed when we had a late arrival in Atlanta. Michael had been sleeping the first leg of the flight, so I didn't notice the inconspicuous change in him. We needed to really hurry if we were to make our connection. However, as we deplaned I could see by his listlessness that was not going to happen. It was reminiscent of the last time we had been in the Atlanta airport. When we got to the correct terminal he was walking at a snail's pace. Was it the encephalopathy at work? I didn't have time to contemplate the question. The only way to be at the gate on time to make our flight was for me to leave him and check us in. I ran ahead, every once in a while stopping and looking back to make sure he was still following me. Why didn't I get a wheel chair? Honestly, it didn't occur to me at the time, nor would I accept the fact that my husband may have needed one.

The agents had just shut the door as I rushed up to the gate. We had missed our connecting plane. There was no point in arguing with them. I turned around and went back to collect my hubby who was still lagging way behind. Together we went to the area for displaced flyers. We approached a different agent with tickets in hand. Even though I tried to intercede, Michael took the lead as he always did with regard to our travels. It was very disconcerting for me when I realized that he wasn't capable of accomplishing that simple task. His speech was slurred as he tried without any success to explain our situation. There is no question that the patient woman behind the desk thought he had been drinking. When it became apparent that he couldn't handle the ticketing himself, I told him to go sit down and that I would take care of it. He obeyed me as if he were a small child. I was on total automatic and did not want to think about what was happening to the man I love.

Six hours later we arrived at our hotel in Rochester exhausted and hungry. As strange as it sounds, I felt better being close to Mayo Clinic than I had felt anywhere in a long time. I desparately needed help with Michael and hoped that wonderful institution would be able to accommodate. I had no idea how tense I had been all day until I was there and able to relax. Originally I hadn't wanted to come. How things had changed in the matter of a few hours. I fell asleep with visions of a drunk husband on a slippery slope weaving in and out of my unconscious mind.

When examined the next morning, Michael was much better. Jack was mostly concerned with the water retention, which had increased not only in the peritoneal cavity, but also in his legs, causing more swelling there as well. When his mental capacity was addressed Michael got extremely agitated again and denied there was a problem, so it was tabled for a while. However, the ascites was such that Jack insisted it be attended to immediately.

Oh boy! Michael was going to be invaded again. Actually, the procedure, known as paracentesis, turned out to be relatively easy. The fluid was extracted from the abdomen using a long needle connected to a device that would pump it out. The doctor eliminated between seven and eight liters of the stuff. When Michael joined me afterwards he was considerably thinner even though his legs were still quite large. He told me it hadn't hurt and the discomfort of feeling bloated along with not being able to breathe well was gone. I hadn't realized how badly the ascites was affecting him until he felt better. We were told the diuretics would have to be increased once more. The fluid accumulation was a strange thing. I don't think either one of us knew quite what to make of it. I for one couldn't understand how there could be such a huge buildup of water in his body in such a short period of time.

All the other appointments were unremarkable. The encephalopathy was finally addressed when Jack and I found time to be alone, as it was evident to both of us that Michael was extremely sensitive concerning that particular topic. He informed me it would probably come back and would be more extreme at times. Then he listed the signs I should look for: fatigue, apathy, irritability, confusion, impaired judgment, inability to concentrate, disorientation and on and on. "You've got to be kidding me!" I moaned out loud. I wanted to believe that once the medications were regulated and the ascites was taken care of, the ammonia would dissipate and stay under control. I definitely wasn't being realistic or pragmatic.

During Michael's scheduled appointment, Jack told us that his liver function was stable, as was the meld score even though the symptoms of liver disease were worse. My thought was that Jack wasn't being as transparent as he could be. It was his nature to try and protect us and I loved that about him, so I let it go. Reigning in my doubts and trying to remain positive was becoming a chore. We traveled home with my thoughts of a slippery slope ever present.

Chapter 10

UNTIL SUDDENLY
Late June 2012

Mayo and the long trip overseas before it had given us few days at home. We were very glad to be back where the island was ours. It was summer, meaning no snowbirds. All medical matters appeared under control for the time at hand. The two of us were relaxed and feeling good. Michael started making plans for the trip of a lifetime we had wanted to take for years: a cruise around the world, due to depart the following January. How bizarre that plan sounds to me now. What was I thinking? I knew Michael had physical, as well as mental challenges. How insane I was to contemplate going away with him for months. Nevertheless, it seemed to be a good juncture in our lives and we were ready to enjoy it. I felt there was no point in thinking about cancer and liver disease when we had so many dreams to live out.

Until suddenly… it began: the slippery slope I had been dreading. In a short period Michael's belly filled with fluid again. I couldn't believe it! The paracentesis at Mayo had only taken place a couple of weeks earlier. We went to see Isaac who told us the draining process needed to be repeated. They took out liters of fluid again. Where was it all coming from? Was it going to be a regular occurrence? We didn't know the answer. If our doctor did, he didn't mention it and as usual I didn't want to ask. Thinking back to that day I realize I was fooling myself once more in thinking everything was eventually going to be fine.

Until suddenly… sometime between 4 and 5 a.m., I was awakened by an exceptionally loud thud. In the quiet of the early morning hours it probably seemed much more explosive that it actually was. As I jumped up and switched on the light in one swift motion, I found Michael lying on the floor, face down at the foot of the bed with his shorts around his ankles and the bench that usually sat there overturned on top of him, obscuring his body. He had obviously fallen when going in or out of the head and was just lying there, not even attempting to get up. What in the world was going on? Was he unconscious? Had he been sleep walking? With a sense of alarm I moved the bench and examined him as best I could. He appeared awake, as his eyes were open, but the glazed look he had told me he was probably unaware of his surroundings. I asked him simply, "What happened?" There was no answer. After further inspecting him, my assessment was that he didn't appear to have hurt himself and wasn't in pain of any kind. As I stood over my husband, he merely looked up at me with a dumb expression on his face, smiling while not saying a word. It took all my strength to finally get him to his feet and pull his underwear up only to have him fall, taking us both down. He had the appearance of being roaring drunk. I deduced it was the encephalopathy. However, it was much worse than the last couple of times it had occurred. Not only could Mickey not stand or talk, he didn't understand anything I was saying; he was totally incoherent and uncontrollable. He kept trying to rise, but couldn't. He tried to walk up the stairs to the galley, but fell backwards repeatedly on me. All the time I was pleading with him to sit or lie down, concerned that he would injure himself. I was completely at my wit's end.

While trying to figure out exactly what to do, a new unwelcome thought invaded my mind: Could something else be wrong? Even though it appeared to be the encephalopathy, my imagination was going wild, as I thought of all the possibilities. I was panicking! I needed help! Without a second thought I had a plan of action. Placing a call to EMS was the only thing to do.

It felt like a very long time, although it was only a few minutes, before an ambulance, fire truck and police car arrived at the quiet dark marina with sirens blaring. Leaving Michael for a moment, I raced to the bow of the boat where I waved the men over to our slip. I was relieved to have the six strong young guys come to my rescue. They wasted no time taking over my charge. Although Michael fought them with what little strength he had, in minutes they had him subdued and hooked up to their equipment as I answered their many questions. After a quick checkup it was agreed that he be taken to Sarasota Memorial Hospital. All of them were needed to carry him through the boat. Once at the outside stairway, they literally passed him from one person to the next until he was down the steps and on the dock where a gurney was waiting.

My mind unleashed a million unwanted scenarios as we raced to the hospital in the ambulance. Throughout the entire time, Michael remained confused and unable to communicate. Once situated in a small ER room, there were more questions I needed to address and many tests to be done. Not only did the doctors have to appraise him physically, they also had to size up his mental capacity. When asked the simplest of questions, like his birthday, he only laughed. He didn't know what year it was or who our president was. When they finished with their assessment and all their tests, the professionals concluded I had been right in the beginning. It was the encephalopathy after all. They assured me that calling EMS was the right move, because left untreated the affliction can cause a coma and be life threatening. That danger was not part of the list I had compiled in my mind regarding the condition of encephalopathy and the word "coma" frightened me half to death, especially since I understood how serious that could be if it happened. I was relieved that there hadn't been anything else wrong and at the same moment shuddered at the thought of what was yet to come.

Once it was concluded that Michael needed to be admitted to Sarasota Memorial Hospital we were assigned to a hospital internist who took over his case from the department head of emergency medicine Dr. Joel Gerber. I gave the new doc all the background info that I had memorized and he called Jack at Mayo Clinic for the rest. Together they decided on a course of treatment. After being in the ER all day my husband was taken to a room. It was good that he was staying in the hospital, as there was no way that I could have taken him anywhere anytime soon in his current state without him killing both of us.

The very next day an uninvited internist appeared in the hospital room. We had used her as our doctor when we first moved to Sarasota, but she hadn't seen either of us in years. I didn't recognize her, nor did I know who she was at first. I guessed that her name must have mistakenly been listed as a contact, because she announced she was the physician of record and was taking over my husband's case. Then without much preamble, she asked Michael if he was on a liver transplant list. I was completely appalled and caught off balance at the mention of a transplant; the prospect, of which had never occurred to either of us. Thankfully my hubby couldn't comprehend much at the time. I, however was aghast. The word "transplant" hadn't come up before and it utterly shocked me. I had never fired a doctor before; I did that day. There was no way Michael was going to have her anywhere near him. He would stay with the hospital internist. After all, he had already coordinated everything with Jack and they had his medical problems under control. Even so, the seemingly tactless doctor had spooked me with her unwanted talk of a liver transplant. Where did that come from? She knew nothing about my husband; he was going to be fine, I told myself, refusing to believe there was a possibility he could be seriously ill.

Michael was hospitalized for a week during that stay. The abdominal fluid was drained again and he was put through millions of tests, one of which showed his kidneys were not functioning properly. A nephrologist was called in to consult on his case because Michael's creatine level was too high. His kidney function needed to be monitored, as the diuretics along with the paracentesis were doing a serious number on them. There was a chance that, if not followed carefully, Michael could go into renal failure. Once again I was in shock as I listened to what could happen to his kidneys. It was so hard to conceive that he could get any worse.

That's when I questioned why his urine was dark orange and not the pale yellow it had always been. I hadn't given it a second thought the past few months as I didn't think it relevant to the alpha-1 antitripsin deficiency. The doctor advised me it was yet another symptom of liver disease.

The nephrologist, together with Isaac, would need to watch his kidneys con-scientiously, as well as all his liver numbers. It seemed like a good plan. We certainly didn't want kidney complications along with the liver disease. As I mentioned before, liver damage can cause low levels of albumin, which is needed for fluid balance, and his level was going down, so they both would also oversee that number too.

During one of the many tests that were done, it was discovered that Michael had fluid accumulation not only in his belly and legs but also in his lungs. It was something else that the doctors were uneasy about, because there was a possibility it could become infected and that would mean more trouble like the development of pneumonia. It reminded me of the pulmonologist at Mayo Clinic long ago who had warned us of impending lung difficulty. I shuddered at the thought.

While he was in the hospital I learned that the amount of ammonia in Michael's body would be tracked on a regular basis by a specific blood test, as that number needed to be watched closely along with the other levels. His was elevated, so an additional drug had been added to Michael's growing number of medications. This one would hopefully contain the encephalopathy. The new med, lactulose, was a sickly sweet syrup that curbed ammonia production, while working as an extremely strong laxative. Simply stated, because his liver couldn't process ammonia, the laxative would help to lower it in his body by forcing it to leave, via his bowels, before it got to his brain. He had to take the ghastly liquid medication several times during the day causing him to poop at least four times a day if it worked properly. Michael really hated the drug, but it did the job. Our life became all about his pooping. As long as he pooped regularly, the encephalopathy would stay in check. I hadn't realized how many bodily functions were related to the liver.

At the end of the week, we were home and pooping. Michael's mental status returned to, what seemed to be on the verge of normal; however, the previous scary week had put me on high alert with reoccurring visions of a liver transplant, coma, renal failure and pneumonia. I realized Michael would need continuous ongoing medical management for I didn't know how long. There was so much to oversee and worry about. My thoughts were ominous as the list of problems continued to grow. I felt as if we were in a free fall without a safety net.

Chapter 11

WHY?
July 2012

The ascites was awful for Michael. It had become a source of extreme discomfort. At first the paracentesis was done just occasionally, but before long we were at the hospital once a week, with liters of the liquid being taken out of the peritoneal cavity every time and it still wasn't happening soon enough for him. He became miserable long before it was time to have it done. With his organs being crowded by the fluid accumulation, and because it was also in his lungs, he developed excessive shortness of breath which was difficult to endure. Just walking was hard for him. A simple thing like eating became a chore and he grew nauseous when he did. He could no longer have regular meals; they had to be quite small because his abdomen was also being crushed by the accumulation of the water. His lower legs turned into "cankles" (swollen or thick ankles) from the fluid dropping down and depositing there. He needed to wear special compression stockings up to his knees to reduce the swelling, which was bothersome given that we live in Florida where it is always quite warm. As for the other symptoms, most of them remained somewhat stable, except for his sallow complexion, which had a significantly more yellowish tinge than even a month earlier and could be especially seen in the whites of his eyes.

With the paracentesis taking place more than weekly, Jack, along with the other doctors, agreed that a procedure called TIPS (transjugular intrahepatic portosystemic shunt) was needed. Jack explained to us over the phone that not only was there a good chance that Michael could develop an infection because the paracentesis was being done so regularly, but there was another risk known as esophageal varices. Blood entering the damaged liver could back up, distending blood vessels in the esophagus and sometimes even in the stomach, which could cause those vessels to bleed. With the TIPS procedure, an artificial shunt would reroute the blood flow to and from the liver, hopefully correcting the problem. A needle would be inserted via the jugular vein in the neck. It would go into the hepatic vein and then the portal vein. An inflatable tipped catheter would serve to bypass blood vessels in the liver, thereby reducing pressure within the portal vein and its branches. It was a lot to take in and sounded menacing to me, more like surgery than a simple procedure, although I wasn't shocked at the time or upset about returning to Mayo Clinic. I only wanted Michael to get better and the TIPS sounded like it would do the job. Jack assured us it wasn't dangerous and would help process the fluid, so it would no longer go into Michael's belly. Therefore, he wouldn't need the paracentesis done and the chance of infection, plus the risk of varices, would be reduced considerably. In addition it would help to stabilize his kidney function. Even though we were hesitant to do another so-called procedure, we agreed to go ahead with it, as not having it done was risky. The only positive aspect was the relief I felt that the ascites would be alleviated. I sort of knew that it was not as easy a fix as I was being told, but didn't contemplate that thought for very long. I trusted that Jack was recommending the best course of action to take regarding Michael's health.

Once again we were heading to Mayo Clinic. Thank goodness Michael tolerated the trip well. Our daughter Amy joined us there. By now I knew our kids didn't trust me to tell them the truth. One reason was that neither Michael nor I chose to talk to them in depth about his liver disease. Anyway, they were probably right not to have confidence in what they were told since I was in Pollyanna land. I think Amy was sent to check out the situation and report to the rest of our family.

As we went to our appointment with Jack, I was in a great mood. The encephalopathy was finally under control now that Michael was pooping routinely. Soon the ascites would be taken care of once the TIPS was done. I thought again that maybe, just maybe, things were getting better for us. Thoughts of our trip around the world edged their way back into my illogically optimistic mind.

Once in Jack's office I realized what a fool I had been. While talking about the TIPS, Jack informed us that there was a possibility the encephalopathy could intensify after the procedure. He then gave us the really bad news. The blood test that had been done that day showed Michael's liver numbers not to be as good as we had expected. His meld score was entering a perilous zone. The Jack who had always been upbeat and positive wasn't there. He did not mince words when he added that, although he wasn't in any crisis at that moment, most patients with that high of a meld score were listed for liver transplant. There was that transplant word again. It debilitated me. Jack continued with the new reality check. Because Michael hadn't been cancer free for five years, he would most likely not be an acceptable candidate for Mayo Clinic's transplant program anyway. He told us that he had made an appointment for him to meet with the liver transplant team regardless of their protocol and that he would use whatever connections he had to get my husband placed on Mayo's list. He thought that maybe they would consider him. The whole conversation shook me up. I didn't want to even reflect upon it, as I refused to believe a liver transplant could be a viable option. I was jolted once more when Michael asked, "What are you telling us Jack? Are you saying I don't have a lot of time left?" When I saw the tears in the eyes of our doctor and good friend, I lost it completely. He acknowledged his answer by nodding his head; he was too choked up to talk. Then he stood, first hugging Michael then me. When he left us alone in the office we held each other and cried. The despair we were both feeling was blatant. Did Jack just tell us that my husband was dying?

When we saw Amy in the lobby she knew immediately something was terribly wrong. It was so very hard to tell her what Jack had said and even harder for her to try to digest the alarming announcement. We were so stunned we couldn't move or talk. After a while we had to reveal the truth to the rest of our family. It was heart wrenching for me to admit Michael was so sick. "How long did he have?" was never answered that day, but the prognosis wasn't good by any stretch of the imagination. Now I understood why Jack never responded when I had asked him, "Is this the beginning of the end?"

One day later we were back at the hospital for the TIPS. After kissing my husband as he was taken away from me for yet another surgical procedure, I sank into a chair and wept, as I had many times before, because I really felt I could be losing him. Amy tried to console me, but no one could have. Finally composed, we talked about what a good father, papa and person he had been throughout his life and that everyone he knew really liked him. We shared how we had always known him to be kind, generous and always willing to help those in need. I remembered him giving money to the homeless and it wasn't uncommon for him to overpay for something, knowing the person selling a product or doing a service really needed the money. I thought how proud I was to be his wife and of course, asked the "why" question as most people do when faced with a frightful situation. Why was this happening to my wonderful man? I felt that in my entire life no one had or ever would love me the way he did. How could I live without that love?

Waiting for Michael while he was getting the TIPS was a nerve-racking time. I was so worried his mind would not be good, that the encephalopathy would be present and maybe worse, that I might not be able to have a meaningful conversation with him. I stood by his bedside when he arrived back in the room, waiting apprehensively for him to speak to me. As I looked at him he looked back up at me from his hospital bed, curiously asking, "Who are you?" I was horror-struck at first and would have been upset if I hadn't seen that little twinkle in his eyes telling me he was playing. It was his personality to joke at a time like that. Realizing he was fine made me furious, but when the doctor came into the room informing us that the TIPS procedure was a success and that the shunt was working perfectly, all was forgiven. The hated ascites was gone, along with the threat of the varices and his mind seemed good. Whew! I felt we had dodged a bullet.

That night our boys, Adam and Darren, came to Rochester. They couldn't stay away, given what we had told them the previous day. They gave us the support that we needed. The next morning Jack came to see Michael. He looked at his numbers from the tests done that morning and was totally amazed at what he saw. The meld score had actually gone down to a more reasonable number and the other results looked good as well. He warned us it was probably temporary, not wanting to get our hopes up, but we were all decidedly encouraged anyway. I was hoping maybe the TIPS was accomplishing more than we had initially been told it would. Immediately my feelings went from being despondent to being hopeful. I wanted so much to envision that my husband was going to be all right that even the slightest bit of positive information had that effect on me.

I was glad Jack got to meet our children and answer their numerous questions. Our boys really gave him the third degree. All of us felt better when he left the room. The day Michael got out of the hospital he was feeling great, so great that our kids started questioning why they had come. The bad tidings from the day before had become a thing of the past. Our thoughts were that the ascites was gone and that Jack had been overly cautious with his talk of a transplant, his prediction about the risk of the encephalopathy increasing and the meld score rising. It was what we all wanted to believe, especially me.

We went out for an enjoyable dinner that night, just like the old days. Michael was back to his old self: fun and lively, ordering everything on the menu. I welcomed the change in him, slowly slipping back to a place where delusion rules. We hadn't had a night like that in a long while. When the kids said their goodbyes the next day none of us could fathom that they wouldn't see the jovial guy of the night before for a very long time to come. I guess I wasn't the only one in denial at that time.

Upon seeing Jack the next day, he informed us he had set up a consultation with the liver transplant team that week. He really wanted us to go, but I had no desire to do so. A transplant, at that point, was well off my radar screen and Michael's too, as he appeared to be doing so well. However, Jack had made the appointment and insisted that we keep it. The minute we arrived at the transplant department I felt uncomfortable and out of place. Many of the people I observed were in wheel chairs and could barely hold up their heads. Michael was nothing like that. We remarked to one another that being there was a total waste of our time. Consequently, when we entered the exam room neither of us took the meeting with the transplant doctors seriously. It was surprising that the two surgeons didn't want to check him over; they only wanted to interview us. We answered questions about our life, offering little information and joked around with them. Not once did either of us ask anything pertinent regarding the liver transplant process. I would say that we were very blasé. Looking back, being notably casual and not caring about the appointment was a mistake, even though I doubt it would have made a difference in their selection. The "cancer free for five years" business stopped them from considering Michael for their list anyway. I didn't really care as I was convinced a transplant was never going to happen. Later that month we got a letter confirming Michael was currently not acceptable for their program. It sounds stupid now, but I was very glad. I didn't want my husband to have to go through such an awful surgery with its months of recovery and plethora of drugs. At the time I was totally convinced he would never need a liver transplant. Still, even though Michael was seemingly better at that point the "why" question continued to plague me. Why was all this happening to such a good man?

Chapter 12

THE DAY FROM HELL

Early August 2012

Michael and I wanted a break from the emotional roller coaster we had experienced at Mayo Clinic, so we decided to take a train to Chicago, spend a night with Sally and Michael and then fly home from there. At the station in Minnesota, we checked our bags and waited for the train to arrive. After hours of biding our time the exceedingly late train appeared and we were on our way. That's when my absent minded lover boy remembered to take his lactulose. I hadn't thought that I needed to remind him, but in retrospect I was dead wrong. Where was it? In his suitcase, in an inaccessible luggage compartment, that's where! Oh well, he would have to take it when we arrived in a few hours. That would work. Or would it? Remember, it's all about the pooping? Well, he hadn't. Was I going to have to start taking care of his meds?

The train ride was tiring for Michael. After we arrived at my sister's house, the four of us went to dinner. He could hardly keep his eyes open. It was a forewarning of things to come, but I refused to recognize the signs. The next day he was still lethargic and had difficulty operating the computer until my sister came to his rescue. That should have been another signal to me that he wasn't all right.

We were due to fly to Tampa that morning, where we had left our car at a hotel parking garage, then drive a little more than an hour home. I couldn't wait to get back where he could rest. Sally drove us to the airport and we made our way through security. My man was slowing down by the minute. I started recognizing the definite presence of encephalopathy. He had been taking his meds on time once we had gotten off the train and according to my calculations he should have been good to go by then, but he wasn't. Watching him sleep on the airplane, I thought maybe he'd be better when we landed. After disembarking the plane in Tampa, all he wanted to do was sit down, but I felt we needed to get on our way. I considered getting a wheelchair for him, but he became belligerent at the suggestion. Without an option I grabbed his hand, pulling him through the airport like I would a difficult 2-year-old. I instantly thought of the ever-present slippery slope again.

I planted the big guy on a chair in the baggage claim area while I collected our suitcases as he looked on. I couldn't help but think of how he had always been in charge and how our roles had been gradually changing. It made me truly gloomy, but there was no time to feel sorry for myself. I got the luggage, wheeled it outside to where the vans going to the hotels were parked and went back to get Michael, who was slouched on a chair. I led him outside, found our driver, and gave him an ample tip. He helped me get Mickey and our bags on and then off the van.

Once at the hotel I deposited my hubby with all of our belongings on a bench under the porte cochere. With money in hand, the valet agreed to help out and watch over him. I gave the man a simple explanation of his condition with instructions to keep checking on him while I got our car. I'm sure he thought Michael had too much to drink, but I was beyond caring what anyone thought. It was quite warm outside, so I attempted to remove the hoodie he was wearing, but he refused to let me touch it, so I left him sleeping next to a family with his hoodie on in the 90 degree weather that he didn't seem to feel. To say the situation was not good would have been an understatement. I had to get him out of there and back home as quickly as possible.

With great haste I headed through the lobby of the hotel to the parking structure, took the elevator and went to the empty space where I remembered parking our car. I thought I knew exactly the spot where it was located, but no, it wasn't there. I proceeded to search the entire level. "OK", I said out loud, because by then I was talking to myself, "Where the hell is it?" I was dripping with sweat as I trudged through several levels of the very hot garage. "It is inconceivable; this can't be happening!" I thought over and over again. There was no time to waste as I was terribly concerned about Michael waiting for me by himself. Could he have somehow moved the car from the original spot the night we checked into the hotel? I tried to recollect what had transpired, but came up blank and I started to get flustered. I had to check on Michael, thinking he must be hot, tired, hungry, thirsty and sick. You name it and I'm sure it went through my agitated brain. I rushed back to the porte cochere where I found him still sleeping. The original family had been replaced by another one, but he was so out of it that he was oblivious to his surroundings.

It occurred to me that there were two parking structures, so just maybe I searched the wrong one. The hotel employee I asked directions of thought I would be better off talking to security after I told her I couldn't find my car. They would have a golf cart and could drive me around to look for it. She directed me to the office, which was located at the far end of one of the parking structures. I did a walk/run to get there. Out of breath, I calmly told the security guard my story, waiting for him to kindly come to my rescue. However, all he did was ask me if I owned a small blue car. When I said yes, he only stared at me and sent me to see his super who was, of course, at the other end of the next parking structure. "Why?" I asked. His lips were sealed. "Did something happen to my car?" No reply from the crusty old guard. Although frustrated, I didn't get angry. I just turned around, doing my walk/run in the opposite direction through the two parking structures, where I found another older crustier guard whose surly disposition was not much different than the first one. As sweetly as I could, I recited my story and asked, "Did something happen to my car?" Only that time I was told to go to the front desk of the hotel. "Could someone please help me!" my mind screamed silently.

The bad news was that I was then almost two hours into the disastrous episode I was living through and nothing positive had happened yet. I turned around, taking another long walk back to the hotel where I checked on sleeping beauty, who was still exactly as I had left him earlier, looking more pallid than he had before. His bench mates had changed once again and he was dozing next to a group of business travelers. My distress intensified as I looked at the scene.

Back inside I found myself in a long line at the front desk. I tried to get one of the bellman to help me speed things along, but that didn't work. With no alternative, I decided to wait patiently. Finally, a pleasant young woman addressed me. I coolly repeated the story of my sick husband and my missing car. After offering her sympathy for my predicament, she asked me if my car was blue. Once again, I asked in a matter of fact manner, "Did something happen to my car?" Her answer was, "I need to get the hotel manager." Now I knew; I didn't have to ask the car question again. Something had definitely happened to my car.

When the manager appeared, he had a very grave look on his face. As I stood in front of him I waited for him to say what I surely didn't want to hear.

Looking down at me, he announced in a scolding tone, "Your car was towed, because it had been partially blocking a pedestrian walkway." I took in the information very stoically while I tried not to burst into tears. Without further comment he abruptly turned me over to the original front desk attendant. She was as nice as she could be, feeling very sorry for me and the state of my affairs. She informed me that my car had been taken several miles away in the opposite direction of our home. I could add another hour to the current fiasco. However, she said she would have the hotel van take us to the lot where it had been towed. "That's nice, maybe our luck is changing", I thought sarcastically.

She then hit me with more unpleasant news; the charge for the tow was $400. In an unperturbed tone, I asked, "Is there anything else?" Thinking, " How could there be?" "Yes!" she answered, "It has to be paid in cash." Wonderful! Before looking for an ATM I checked on Michael again, who was still looking ghastly and then off I went to get the cash. I wasn't sure we even had that much money available in our checking account. Michael always took care of our money matters. Once more, I was sad for a moment, our financial situation was all new to me. I started to feel helpless. "What ifs" flooded my head. "Pull yourself together!" I thought, as I willed my mind to get back down to business. The money was there plus some extra just in case, so I collected it from the machine and went outside to wait with Michael for the van that would take us to our car. I needed to get him home so I could take care of him or maybe take him to the hospital. As I was daydreaming of a trip to the ER, my front desk lady appeared looking very sheepish. The van was not going to be able to pick us up for more than an hour. It was beyond belief! Agitation had now turned to resignation. With a fake smile, I asked her to call us a taxi.

The cab was going to be a small fortune. It was a good thing I had taken out some extra cash. As we drove through Tampa the area was getting more run-down by the mile. We finally got dropped off at the tow yard, which I couldn't refer to as a garage because it was a field overgrown with weeds, and with all types of unusable vehicles scattered here and there. To top it off, we were in the seediest of the seedy parts of town and it was getting dark. I left my sleepy husband sitting on our bags in the front of the dilapidated building, knowing he would not be able to maneuver the stairs to the office. The hefty, heavily made-up lady in charge gingerly took my money then asked for the registration for the car. "No registration, no keys" was the rule. I needed the keys to get the registration. It was in the car; I wasn't in the habit of carrying it around with me. After an idiotic conversation, she finally agreed to let a tattooed, bearded, dirty, smelly wonder of the male species go with me to the car to get the registration. It took me some time to find where Michael kept the car papers. Once I had the registration in hand, I presented it to the boss lady and she finally gave me the keys. The greasy man was pleased with the tip I gave him and helped me put Michael and the suitcases in the car. We were finally on our way. The whole calamitous situation had taken over four hours and we still weren't home.

As I drove through the darkened streets of Tampa I, of course, had to navigate through a downpour. Nothing was easy that day. The ride was much longer than usual, especially with no one to talk to, as Michael was dead to the world again. That's when I started to think. When did he take his medicine last? He's supposed to poop four times a day. Did he poop today? Does he need some water? Does he need to eat something? How was I going to get him on the boat, as his walking was questionable? What about our luggage? We've been away; is there food at home? Should I just give up and take him directly to the ER? Wouldn't that be the best thing to do? It certainly was a reasonable thought. I couldn't turn it off; it went on and on.

I formulated a game plan. Stopping at the grocery store, I parked in front and left Michael in the car. He was in such bad shape by then I knew he wouldn't want to get out anyway. Inside I purchased water with a snack and took it out to him. Back in the store, I gathered some bare necessities. When I got to the car he hadn't touched any of his water or food, causing my worry to escalate. Should I just go to the ER? It was definitely a feasible choice and I had learned from the past it would be much easier giving the hospital staff the responsibility of managing his health rather than attempting to do it myself. In the end my heart told me that I alone needed to take care of my husband. I really didn't know if I could, but I wanted to give it a shot, so I decided to go directly home and talk to Jack. Hopefully I wouldn't have to call for EMS in the middle of the night.

By the time I got to the marina it was well after their closing time and there were no dock hands to help me, so I elected to get Michael on the boat first and contemplate what to do about the bags later. Walking him on the narrow dock was no easy job, with him staggering all over the place, but I steered him down the middle and managed to keep him from falling into the murky water. As we slowly made our way, I looked from boat to boat for some sign of life. All of a sudden there he was, my knight in shining armor. I knew he would come to my rescue. CJ captains a neighboring boat and lucky for me he was working that night. He knew by looking at us that something was very wrong. After I explained what had happened he took over, helping me get Michael on the boat, then retrieving the rest of our luggage from the car and taking it into our stateroom before he went on his way.

Just as I was getting settled, the electricity went off, leaving us with no air conditioning or light in the sweltering heat. I called CJ but he didn't answer. The newest crisis would have to wait. I got out our portable lanterns and called Jack. As usual he calmed me down. He told me to increase the lactulose right away to every two hours. If that didn't work I would have to drive my guy to the hospital or call EMS. Having to take the extra dose of medication got

Michael very peeved. I forced him and then made him a peanut butter and jelly sandwich. He sat with his arms dangling at his sides as I fed him in the light of the lanterns, all the while holding back my tears. The scene was heart wrenching for me. Jack's words about his meld score and the encephalopathy and all his other symptoms preyed upon my mind. "Is this the beginning of the end? Are we coming to the bottom of that slippery slope?" I thought over and over again.

I had no time to reflect, as the power was next on my agenda. I called CJ again and this time he answered. He was back from dinner and came over immediately. We were in the process of having our generators overhauled, so they could not be used as a back up. He would have to find the source of the power problem, which he deduced was in the control panel. Together we phoned Patrick, who maintains our boat, and he walked CJ through the steps to get the electricity functioning again. Soon it was up and running and things were looking up. The air and lights were on and, thank goodness, Michael was pooping. He seemed better already.

I left him sleeping in the main salon and went down to our stateroom to get us unpacked and organized. It wasn't long before the power was off again. When I got upstairs I found my ditzy Captain Mickey laboring at the control panel in the dark, trying to fix it. I couldn't believe what I was witnessing. Even though he wasn't as wacky as he'd been earlier that day, he was far from adept enough to address an electrical issue. It took some time to pull him away, but I eventually coaxed him back to the couch, after which I went looking for CJ, but he had left the dock for the night. I tried to call Patrick, but he didn't answer. Remembering the marina had an emergency number I called it. The young woman on duty came right away. She didn't have a clue as what to do, so she called the manager of the marina who doubled as a captain. He had me try everything he could think of, but doing it over the phone was impossible.

In the meantime I started packing an overnight bag. There was no way we could stay on the boat in the oppressive heat.

Just as I was getting ready to leave, Patrick finally called back. Michael, while working on the boat's control panel, had haphazardly changed the switches, causing more of a mess than we already had. After going through numerous exercises with the various controls, Patrick had me take several pictures of the panel with my cell phone. I sent him all the views and he instantaneously saw where the problem was. With his help I was able to get the system up and working again. I prayed it would stay on. Taking Michael to a hotel in the middle of the night after the terrible day he had would not be the best thing for him. He needed to be in bed right away.

Upon returning to the salon I expected to find Michael snoozing. Instead he had the remote control for the TV in his hand and was in the process of wreaking havoc on that. Before I could stop him it was dead. Oh well, nothing could faze me at that point.

It was late and time for us to turn in. Once in our stateroom it wasn't surprising Michael got hold of the remote there and screwed up that TV. I was so tired I didn't care. That day had truly been the day from hell. I was done, and didn't want to deal with anything else, especially what was in store for us down the road. I feared that what I had experienced the last 24 hours could be a sample of the chaos the future held.

Upon awaking the next morning I found the TV in the galley wasn't working either. Hmmm . . .

Chapter 13

ADJUSTING TO OUR NEW EXISTENCE
August and Early September 2012

It took Michael some time to recover from his latest bout of encephalopathy. In fact, although I didn't want to admit it, he was really much worse after the day from hell. There were not any great days anymore. The encephalopathy was always present in different degrees. I tended to rate him daily on how bad he was, with "not bad" meaning he was better at that time. When I think back, it's hard for me to realize what we lived through during that wretched juncture in our lives.

On a not bad day, even though Michael still showed some mild signs of encephalopathy, he was able to drive short distances, go out to lunch or dinner, go to the fitness center for a light workout and watch a movie, which was relaxing for me because I could lose myself for a few hours. He would take care of professional concerns, talk to friends and we could have meaningful conversations while making some decisions. In August he was still trying to handle our finances and deal with his various business interests. I could leave him alone for short periods without worrying and he would be fine.

One day that all changed. I left him at home and walked to the fitness center. He was to drive the two miles later in the morning and pick me up. After I'd been there for a while I saw him come in. It was obvious by his demeanor and stagger that he was not doing well. When I looked out at the parking lot and saw our car parked in the middle of the driving lane with a significant dent in the fender I knew I was right. No more driving for him as of that day, which caused a continuous dispute between us. I didn't want to know that he was declining, but there came a point when I couldn't deny it.

It was about that time when Michael's thinking process along with his memory became significantly more affected. He handled it by pretending he was all right. If I so much as suggested that he wasn't mentally competent he would become very contentious. I tried to tell him on a bad day not to talk business with anyone, but the one thing that hadn't left him was his stubborn streak. When he would call his attorney, accountant or other business associates, he sounded confused and couldn't remember the simplest of things. It was so hard to watch. He would go on and on with meaningless chatter, sounding totally stoned. I would try to give a heads up to the unsuspecting person who would be the target of his chitchat. Almost everyone we knew, especially our family, understood about Michael's unstable health, but for the unwarned caller, it was startling.

It was particularly unsettling for those who hadn't seen him in a long time to observe Michael's physical state, as his condition continued to rapidly decline. The muscle loss had left him looking feeble and weak. He couldn't walk straight. In fact, he shuffled his feet while taking very tiny steps and his head hung forward, looking down. I'm sure he was afraid of falling, for he had become more unbalanced. Upon looking at him, you couldn't help but notice his eyes because they tended to bulge. His mouth would sag open and sometimes his tongue would hang out. It was impossible to believe the jaundice could intensify, but it did. I remembered the pity I saw on the faces of friends when Michael had been diagnosed with pancreatic cancer. I hated that look! It had torn me apart then and it was happening all over again with the symptoms of his liver disease.

As Michael's intellectual capacity worsened, our finances became an overwhelming problem for me. After getting married I had gladly let him take over all our banking and bill paying. Being a controlling man he would have it no other way, but because of the encephalopathy I became troubled that he was muddling everything up. If his desk was disorganized before he became ill, afterward it became a disaster. I knew I had to get my arms around the potential quagmire, but was so afraid of hurting his feelings. I would ask him for information regarding our various accounts and got little from him except discombobulation. As a precaution I gave our banker a preemptive call. I dove into the computer when Michael was sleeping, trying to figure out our banking, credit cards and investments. Needless to say, they were in the disorganized state I had expected. He had changed his passwords, probably because he couldn't recall the originals. When I tried a few times I would get booted out and couldn't access the accounts. Then I was automatically referred to the many security questions. One question in particular really stumped me. "Where does your father live?" Well, his dad had lived in Detroit, but it could have also been Oak Park or even Michigan. Oh no! That's not what my honey wrote down. It was "heaven"! That gave me a good laugh when I really needed it.

His equilibrium continued to diminish due to the encephalopathy. I was afraid he'd fall off the dock or down the stairs in the boat, so I was always watching where he was going. Once in a while he would leave without telling me, and I would be a nervous wreck as I searched all over for him. At that point I started looking for a condo or apartment to rent just so I could keep him out of danger and free from any unnecessary harm. Fortunately his days of wandering off didn't last too long.

As the liver disease progressed, it wasn't advisable to leave Michael alone anymore. Consequently, when I would have to do an errand, like going to the grocery store, we would go together. I would help him down the dock and into the car, locking his seat belt for him. It was as if I was caring for a toddler. I would take him to the front of the building, drop him off at a chair, go in, get him a drink, and then park the car. As I left him I would say, "Don't you move! Stay right here until I get back!" Actually, I knew he wouldn't leave because the encephalopathy caused him to be unsure of his surroundings and he wouldn't know where to go anyway, as he was constantly getting lost. Upon my return he was always there waiting and watching for me just like a child would do. Sometimes I would leave him in the car with the window down and the door locked because he couldn't figure out quite how to unlock it. Trying to protect him became my life's mission.

In August, Michael still had many days that were not bad, but when September arrived, the "bad days" really started to escalate. His listlessness and apathy were increasing at a alarming tempo. On a typical day he would wake up, have breakfast and fall asleep on the couch in a matter of minutes. He couldn't leave the boat or do the simplest of tasks. Wherever he was, napping was not problematic. He would drift off in the middle of a conversation. His health had deteriorated to the point that many days I had to feed him, help him wash, brush his teeth and assist him with other various grooming and personal needs. Those were the saddest days of all for me. He had never been a good sleeper at night and always needed sleeping pills. But during that period he would get into bed early without watching TV, which was so unusual for him, and go the entire night barely moving. When my kids were babies I became a light sleeper. The slightest sound from them triggered my mind to come alive. It was exactly the same for me then. I always woke up several times to check on him. It was strange; I used to get irritated when he would wake me up in the middle of the night to keep him company, but now I craved those nights. I wanted all his little annoying habits back in my life.

Talking to Jack or the other doctors really didn't help, as there was nothing they could do except adjust Michael's meds from time to time. We did talk of reversing the TIPS, for it was determined to be the cause of the increase in the encephalopathy, but to do so would definitely result in the ascites coming back and that could be a danger to him. For the moment, it was the status quo.

I always tried not to think about what had happened to our life or what lay ahead of us, but at night when I got into bed, thinking was all I could do. And, of course, praying: praying my husband would come back to me. Some nights I would hold on to him and cry, although he didn't even know I was there. I missed Michael so very much it hurt all the time. I kept hoping he would get better as time went by, but that wasn't in the cards for him. Adjusting to our new existence was one of the hardest challenges of my life.

Chapter 14

WRONG AGAIN

September 2012

*T*houghts of traveling the world were a very distant memory. We both loved the adventure of a long journey, but there was no way we could even get on a plane to visit our kids. The next best variation we could muster in our otherwise mundane existence was driving 20 minutes to my sister and brother-in-law's condo on Anna Maria Island, which overlooked the beautiful beach. If nothing else, it would be a welcome novelty for us, as there was little else we could do.

After driving the short distance we settled into the roomy condo. Having a new routine with a different setting was good for both of us. Michael really enjoyed the breeze while sitting on the balcony overlooking the Gulf of Mexico. He couldn't actually go into the Gulf or even the swimming pool for that matter, but looking at it gave him great pleasure. Having a real kitchen instead of the small galley that I had on the boat gave me the opportunity to cook some substantial meals for him. He needed to put some weight on his skinny frame. It seemed a good change for us. When I look back at that time I can see we were in flux, waiting for something to happen, not knowing exactly what to expect, but knowing without a doubt that there was more adversity heading our way.

I guess it shouldn't have been a surprise when early one morning Michael hit the slippery slope again. He stood to get out of bed and almost fell as he started to walk. Taking one look at his bulging eyes and the befuddled look on his face was all I needed to know that he was in the midst of a full-blown attack of encephalopathy. I tried to talk to him, although I knew from past experience he couldn't speak or understand anything I would say; he just gave me his silly sweet smile. I helped him into the bathroom because I knew that's where he was headed. When I tried to get him to sit on the toilet he became as stiff as a board and remained right where he was standing no matter how I pushed or pulled him. Before I was aware of what was happening or could do anything about it, he had lost all control of his bodily functions. As if that wasn't enough, he started vomiting uncontrollably. The three "p's" hit him all at one time; peeing, pooping and puking. My poor husband! At least he wasn't aware of what was happening. As for me, I was flabbergasted, in a state of total shock and frozen in one spot. I just stared at him, unable to move. He was the epitome of the worst catastrophe anyone could begin to imagine. It was a sight I don't think I will ever forget. For a moment I was at a loss as what to do.

Without a single doubt in my head I knew I had to call EMS. The well-being of Michael was foremost in my mind and he was in grave danger of falling. There was no way I could take care of him by myself; he had gone beyond being manageable. However, before I placed the call I had to get him cleaned up, as I cared for his dignity. I tried as hard as I could to get him into the shower, but again he wouldn't budge from the stance he had taken. Without another option, I washed him as he stood in his own mess while I sobbed without restraint. I didn't have to hold it back. With the encephalopathy erupting in his head he had no idea how emotionally wrought I was. When I finished my task it required all my strength to drag him back to the bedroom. It was like pulling a stubborn mule and it took some time for us to travel the short distance. When I finally got him there I merely shoved him back onto the bed where he collapsed, immediately falling into a deep sleep. While he lay there, I dressed him as best I could, since he was dead weight, and then called EMS. Within a few minutes I heard the welcome sound of the sirens.

I already knew the drill and was ready when my saviors arrived at the condo with all their gear. The relief I felt as they took over was on a grand scale. The adrenaline rush that had been fueling me suddenly vanished as they assumed responsibility for my spouse. The medics readily accepted the diagnosis of encephalopathy that I had given them, in writing, from Mayo Clinic, as they took vitals and started IVs. Even though Sarasota Memorial Hospital wasn't the closest hospital, they agreed to take him there. His life was not in danger and he had been admitted there before with the same set of symptoms. Shakily, I agreed to follow them in my car.

I was numb as I sat in the ER at Michael's bedside, too numb to make the calls I knew I had to make to our kids and family. Michael, on the other hand, was in la la land. The only reaction he had to the simplest questions was laughter. When I told him if he didn't give me a urine sample they were going to insert a catheter in him, he became hysterical as if it were the funniest thing he had ever heard. Even though I didn't feel like it, I found myself laughing along with him. Well, that was better than the alternative.

Being at Sarasota Memorial surrounded by the staff that I had come to know made me feel better. Joel Gerber, the very experienced emergency room doc, and his wife Jeanne, a manager of nurses, were there for us again. It was the second time Michael received their care and I felt their compassion. Joel saw that Michael was too unbalanced mentally and physically to go home, so later in the day he was admitted into the hospital. "Just for a day or two, until he was stable," I was told.

One day turned into two, two into three and so on. All in all, we were there for well over a week. Michael was so amiable and defenseless during his stay that the nurses fell in love with my man-child. When I would leave for the day, they would put him on what he called "lock down," meaning they would arm his bed with an alarm. That way he couldn't get up without the staff being alerted. Can you believe, he paid no attention to it? If he awoke in the middle of the night, he just got right up without a care for the other patients asleep on his floor and let the alarm blast away, causing the nurses within hearing distance to come running. One night, I was informed, he got out of the bed so many times that they finally put him in a wheel chair and brought him to the nurses' station where he proceeded to tell them dirty jokes all night. They thought he was very funny and cute. Part of it was the encephalopathy and part of it was just Mickey being Mickey.

Another wonderful caregiver was Aida Samson, the PA affiliated with Isaac's office. She came to see Michael every day, giving him the very best of her expertise. She was never in a hurry and always had a kind word for both of us. Aida even gave me her personal cellphone number in case I needed her. I felt so fortunate to have her caring for Michael.

While he was in the hospital, my phone would ring nonstop with family and acquaintances wanting to know how he was doing. It was tiring for me to contend with all the questions that I didn't want to answer. Our well-meaning friends would stop by to visit us. Although I loved having the company, it was hard for me to observe the way they looked at Michael. They were frightened for him and felt sorry for both of us. Their visits only served to make me more depressed than I already was.

Throughout the stay in the hospital Michael was given a multitude of tests; nevertheless, there was nothing new to report. Thank goodness that, since the TIPS procedure, his kidney function had normalized. The docs called Jack to confer and the conclusion was to adjust his meds once again. Jack was a firm believer that the more Michael pooped, the less encephalopathic he would be, so his dose of the laxative was increased. It ended up being both bad and good for him, because when he had the encephalopathy he became incontinent, so getting his dose just right was a necessary chore.

The other issue was that the stay in the hospital had left him excessively weak and even more unstable on his feet, so physical therapy was ordered as part of his daily routine. With their methods of rehabilitation, he would be using the muscles he would need when he was ultimately released. Although it drained him, he was a trooper and worked with them as best he could. He wanted very badly to go home with me and would do anything they asked of him to achieve that goal.

Every day when I got to the hospital I thought we'd be able to leave, but the doctors didn't want to discharge Michael until he was walking reasonably well, able to manage stairs and pooping great. And he, of course, needed to be mentally alert and not a danger to himself or to me. Finally, the time came for his release. I was so relieved to be taking him out of the hospital. All of our belongings were still at the beach condo, so that was where I was going to take him. The fridge was already stocked and everything was ready for Mickey's homecoming. I couldn't wait to get back him back there to recuperate. He had a big smile on his face when I came to pick him up that morning and was so happy. Once more I thought that he was going to be relatively fine. Wrong again!"

Chapter 15

PRETENDING NOT TO KNOW

September 2012

I happily departed the hospital for the condo on the beach with Michael in tow, along with a completely distorted view of reality. On the way to Anna Maria Island, I needed to stop at the pharmacy for some new prescriptions that had been called in. Leaving him in the car, I went inside the drug store to fetch the meds. A few minutes later I returned to find my hubby covered in vomit. I stood with the car door open taking in the scene, not wanting to believe what I was witnessing. He told me sheepishly that when he started to feel sick he couldn't get the car door open. I felt as if I were with a small boy who thought he was about to be scolded. "No worries, baby, I'll take care of it," I calmly assured him, although not feeling that way at all. Eventually, I went into action mode. I ran back into the store, purchased some wipes and got a clean shirt from the bag in the trunk. Then I cleaned him up while he sat in the front seat. When that was done, I called the doctor's office. Isaac had examined Michael that very morning before we left the hospital. I was sure I would be headed back to Sarasota Memorial, however it was Friday afternoon and he was not available. The nurse told me not to worry, that Michael had probably been carsick as a result of the encephalopathy and being in the hospital so long. I wanted to accept that explanation, but didn't. Truthfully, I was afraid to be alone with my husband and I felt inclined to take him back to Sarasota Memorial Hospital. Now I understand that I instinctively knew what was best for his well-being. Not taking him to the hospital was a bad move. I should have paid attention to my intuition.

The rest of the ride to the beach went smoothly. Step by step we managed the stairs up to the condo without a hitch, just as we had been instructed to do by the physical therapy tech. Once there, Michael settled on the couch and fell sound asleep immediately, while I busied myself making him dinner. I figured he'd be out for an hour. After an hour and a half I woke him up, thinking immediately that he wasn't feeling good again, but put that thought in the back of my mind for another one, deciding he was just tired from the long day.

He didn't want to eat or leave his place on the couch. With some coaxing I got him to sit at the table for dinner, where his arms hung limply at his sides and his mouth hung open exposing his tongue, while his head swayed to and fro. I had been so excited that very morning with the anticipation of his coming home after such a long hospitalization. A few hours later I felt totally conquered, as I observed the wonderful man in front of me. "Please, not again!" I prayed. He had been pooping great. Didn't Jack and all the other doctors tell me that as long as he pooped regularly he'd be fine? Something wasn't right. After all, he'd just been released from the hospital. I was distraught as I pulled up a chair to the table and fed him like a child once more. He wouldn't eat much and just wanted to go back to the couch, so I gave in. After a short time I got him into bed; he was only sleeping anyway.

During the night I automatically woke up several times to do my check on Michael, disregarding the fact that he had stirred less than usual. He was still sound asleep as I crept out of the room the next morning. When it was time for him to take his meds, I had to wake him. Back in the bedroom I noticed for the first time that it wasn't just that he hadn't changed positions that was odd; he was also very still and his chest was barely moving, causing my heart to palpitate. I said his name then shook him gently. No response! I raised my voice and shook him harder. Nothing! Suddenly I found myself screaming his name over and over as pure panic and hysteria took over. Still nothing! I was crying and yelling as I came to the realization that he was unconscious and at once thought that he may be in a coma. For a split second I imagined the very worst: my husband was dying. Trembling with fright, all I wanted to do was escape the terrifying nightmare I was in. Then the adrenaline rush I experience during a crisis took hold. Whipping the pillow out from under his head, I remembered my Red Cross training and prepared him for CPR. I felt his pulse; it was there but weak and thready. I checked his breath; it was there but shallow. "Thank God he's alive!" I thought. Then I called EMS without taking my eyes off of him. I answered the operator's many questions. The whole time I was ready to do CPR if need be.

Soon there was that welcome sound of the sirens screaming my name as the ambulance arrived. The demeanor of the medics was totally different than the other occasions when I had called them. There was an urgency that hadn't been there on their previous runs. It scared the hell out of me! They took one look at Michael, pushed me aside, and went to work on him. As the medics took out their CPR equipment, I couldn't help but notice that the electric shock paddles were front and center. They first hooked up their EKG machine and started an IV, after which there was more harried prep. When the guys were done with their assessment, they carried him down the two flights of stairs. It was no easy feat, as the staircase was quite narrow and a stretcher would not fit. They had him sitting up with straps up and down his body to keep him from toppling over. His head fell forward as he was still totally unconscious and remained that way as they put him in the ambulance.

At that point I handed them the letter from Mayo Clinic describing their diagnosis of encephalopathy. I also gave them his release papers from the day before. I explained that he had just been in Sarasota Memorial Hospital and that I thought his medical situation was related to the encephalopathy. I wanted him back at that hospital where they were familiar with his case, and I had friends on the staff. That's when the lead paramedic hit me with a zinger. He stated that Michael was displaying all the signs of a stroke and there was no way they could risk taking him all the way to Sarasota. There was a closer hospital and that's where they were going, no discussion. How could they determine he had a stroke when he was unconscious and non-responsive? I was aghast and stunned at the thought of a stroke, not believing what I had just been told. Of course, I instantly acquiesced, as there was little else I could do and I was so afraid they were right or that he may be in a coma. In a matter of minutes we were off, racing down the empty streets with sirens piercing the quiet of the early morning hours.

Being a positive person, I usually stop myself from thinking negative thoughts. Nevertheless, on the ride and later in the ER waiting area, I was entertaining premonitions of the very worst scenario. Once at the hospital, I was told by the front desk that I couldn't see Michael until the doctors called from the back of the ER where they had him hidden, doing I couldn't imagine what to him. I felt utterly helpless as I waited. I cried and cried for him and for myself. The nurse tried talking to me, but there was nothing that could assuage my pain. Soon she took pity on my situation and forsook protocol, leading me into the hospital's "no-fly zone."

When I got to Michael's bedside he was still unconscious, but I talked to him anyway, telling him that he was OK. When did I ever learn to be such a good liar? The one thing I didn't want to do was to give up hope. We would get through the latest calamity, I told both of us.

After scores of tests, which wouldn't have had to be done had we gone to our Sarasota hospital, a very curt doctor came into the room. He informed me that although some tests were pending, he didn't feel Michael had a stroke and he wasn't in a coma. That brought on a big sigh of relief, but what now? He said he would wait for more test results before coming to the conclusion that the encephalopathy had caused Michael's episode that day.

When I had first arrived at the godforsaken hospital, I had asked that Sarasota Memorial Hospital be called. I gave them the name of Michael's attending doctor there and Joel's name, expecting someone to phone them. After all, he had just been released from there the day before. They would surely want to know what his status had been when he had left the other hospital's care. That was not done. Once again I made the very same request and also asked him to call Isaac's office. The ER doctor told me abruptly he was not going to place the calls and that he was admitting Michael for yet more tests and observation. I told the doctor, "That is not what I want." He told me that it wasn't up to me. At that time I didn't have the wherewithal or energy to be assertive and argue my case. "What is that about? Money?" I thought to myself. I felt totally defeated, but even so, I pulled myself together and called my doctors at Sarasota Memorial. They both called me back, agreeing Michael should be back at their hospital, but because the current hospital hadn't released him, their hands were tied and due to the fact it was late, there was little that could be done until morning. It sounded like hospital politics to me. Frustrated, I resigned myself to address the problem of moving Michael the next day.

Once he started to become conscious, Michael was taken upstairs in that awful hospital to an awful room to get equally awful care. We had spent the entire day in the ER and by the time we reached the hospital floor, it was dark. I stood in the hall next to the gurney, drained, as the nurses and attendants laughed and carried on their nonsense behind the desk. I had no patience for that crap. My husband needed to get into a room and have something to eat. More importantly, he hadn't taken his meds all day. After they finally got him into a bed, I noticed he had wet himself. When I went to get his nurse I was informed she was on break and Michael would have to wait. "Break? Give me a break," I thought. Wasn't there anyone else who could have helped? I guess not, so I took care of him myself. I was becoming more infuriated by the minute. All I could think about was getting him out of that disgusting hospital.

By 8 p.m., Michael was only semi-conscious and only semi-aware of what was going on, so I was taken aback when he simply and very seriously pleaded, "Please don't put me in a nursing home." It was one of the most despairing moments I have ever had in my life. How could he think that I would do that? My fearful, sensitive husband was afraid I didn't want to take care of him anymore. I looked at my defenseless man as I gave him my word: "Never, not ever will that happen!" It took all my strength to stay composed. Anyway, that appeased him for a while. However, it was on his mind, even though I tried to reassure him time and time again in the days to come that taking care of him was what I wanted to do. Where did he get such a depressing idea?

Just when I thought the day couldn't get any worse, a slovenly looking physician who smelled of cigarettes showed up to do an evaluation of Michael. My pattern had always been to stay during such exams. Not that time. I left the room and paced the halls trying to get my thoughts together, having no desire to hear what he had to say. Sometime later the doctor found me and straightforwardly asked, "Why isn't your husband at Sarasota Memorial Hospital? I see he's been recently discharged from there. If he stays here he will have to endure all the same testing that he must have already had there." I wanted to say, but only thought, "Duh?" Instead I simply told him that's what I had wanted from the beginning. He simply replied, "Why don't you just leave with him? Put him in your car and go there." Finally, something made sense to me. Of course I can do that. This is a free country, isn't it? Great idea! I found Nurse Ratched and told her I was taking my husband out of the hospital that night and that I needed a wheelchair. The unconscionable woman unceremoniously told me, "You can take him wherever you want, but no one here will help you get him out of bed and put him in a wheelchair and no one here will help you get him into your car!" Talk about being absolutely crushed! There was no way I could move him by myself. He was still just barely conscious and couldn't even stand up.

Checking on Michael, I knew that he was still incoherent, although content and safe, so I left him to find a quiet place to make my calls to family. After talking to our kids I realized how foolish I had been in not calling a private ambulance to move him earlier in the day. I always go by the rules and hadn't thought of that option. Adam volunteered to handle it for me. Within a half hour he had arranged for an independent transport company to come in the morning to retrieve Michael and take him to where he should have been all along, Sarasota Memorial Hospital.

The next morning Michael was pretty much awake, enough to tell me he wanted out of the hospital, that during the night a nurse had yelled at him when he accidentally wet himself again. I had told the nurse to put a diaper on him the night before, but she obviously hadn't done that. Taking him back to Sarasota was definitely the right move. When the ambulance arrived we were ready to go. Upon leaving, the looks and sneers of the staff made me feel as if I were a criminal or a traitor. I walked alongside the gurney holding my husband's hand as I took him away from that hellhole of a hospital without signing him out. I promised both of us that it was the last time they would ever see us there. He was loaded into the ambulance and traveled alone with the medics, as I followed in my car. Since Michael was still pretty goofy, I wasn't surprised to hear that he had begged them to stop on the way for a Dairy Queen. He was so comical during any incidence of encephalopathy that I had to laugh.

Off we went to Sarasota Memorial Hospital where I knew the care would be exemplary. I felt confident that Michael was going to recover. What was I pretending not to know?

Chapter 16

AN HONEST DOSE OF REALITY
September 2012

There are different ways patients enter a hospital. They can come in the front door because a doctor has admitted them for treatment or a procedure; they can walk into the ER when sick or injured; or they can arrive by a city ambulance. Michael's entry was none of the above that day nor was it conventional. In fact, they didn't quite know what to do with him when he arrived by private transport, mostly because he had left the other hospital without being discharged and patients that appear the way he did usually have already been admitted into the hospital prior to their arrival. The staff in the ER couldn't turn him away because he had just been in their hospital, and more importantly, he was far too sick. I found Joel as soon as I arrived. With the compassion that he always showed, he took over and I was able to find some solace for the first time in 48 hours. Soon Michael was in a bed being evaluated for the umpteenth time.

Amy arrived that afternoon and I was comforted by having her there with me. The time for trying to handle Michael's health by myself was over. There was no more flying solo for me. I needed help; I needed my family.

In Michael's ER room I was encouraged that he was completely conscious after the horrendous crisis he had endured the day before. In fact, he was so animated I didn't realize how bad the encephalopathy was. Upon looking at him more closely I saw he was crazier than he had ever been, and any advancement he'd made during his time in physical therapy was gone. Even though he was somewhat improved he could barely sit, let alone walk. He was almost completely bedridden. Then there was his talking. He was slurring his words while saying such gibberish that no one, not even me, could understand him. With garbled speech, over and over, he kept telling anyone who would listen that he wanted "yogi". We finally figured out he was having a craving for yogurt, but he was asking for it while sitting on a commode pooping in the middle of his tiny room with the curtains partially open and two female nurses in attendance. Mickey showed not the slightest sign of embarrassment. He had no concern whatsoever about his current situation.

Once more, my guy spent the entire day in the ER. Later he was admitted to a temporary floor for observation, as the doctors were hoping to get him up and out as soon as possible. There was not much they could do for him anyway. His room happened to be across the hall from where the medications were dispensed, but he thought it was a store and that the packages of meds the nurses kept picking up were food, like ice cream and snacks. Thus, he was constantly trying to get out of bed and "go shopping." As I said before, he was acting like a looney tune.

After a couple of days it was evident Michael was taking a lot longer to recover from his latest setback than originally thought. There was no chance that in his current state he could be released from the hospital any time soon and finally he was taken to what was becoming his hospital floor. All the nurses and aides welcomed him back. During that period the readjusting of his meds and endless blood tests continued. There was nothing pressing about his care. They just wanted to get him regulated enough to go home.

When the Jewish holidays arrived, I knew Michael had hoped to go to services. That was an impossibility, so I had requested a rabbi visit us, but as the day wore on it didn't seem that was likely to happen. Then late afternoon the first night of Rosh Hashana, a rabbi knocked on our door and asked if we'd like to pray with him. The wonderfully religious man, Rabbi Brenner Glickman, had brought along prayer books. He proceeded to create a meaningful short service, shofar and all. Afterwards, Michael, Amy and I, along with the rabbi, held hands as he said a prayer for Michael's wellness. Needless to say, there wasn't a dry eye in the small room, as the whole experience was so emotionally draining. Before the rabbi left, he handed me two prayer books suggesting we should use them in the days to come and that when Michael was well we could return them. I hoped that day would eventually happen. I was so very touched by his generosity, as I knew Michael would be one day if we made it through that trying period. The rabbi had uplifted our spirits and reminded us of the power of prayer. He gave us faith that Michael would ultimately regain his health — faith that we surely needed.

The staff had all grown fond of Mickey and loved coming into his room to talk. The nurses and aides fought to have him as a patient. For them it was like ministering to a little boy in a 6-foot body. His doctors liked his company too, and would sit in his room and chat. Even though he was batty, he was still good to be around when he could talk. He, of course, had nicknamed all of them. One in particular, Dr. Bradd Kaplan, was a favorite. Michael called him "Big Dog" because of his stature. He couldn't walk by the room without my hubby yelling out at the top of his lungs, "Big Dog". When a smaller doc replaced him, the new one became known as "Little Dog".

In the interim, Michael was losing control of his bodily functions more and more often. It was additional evidence of his decline. As usual, I tried to nullify what was happening to him by explaining it away, so I would say he had an accident, as if it was something that was likely not to present itself again. The days he wore adult diapers were extremely disconcerting. Even though I knew that the aides put them on for his comfort and cleanliness, I felt it would cause him great humiliation. I was very wrong. The only concern he ever showed was one day when he asked me, "What is this I have on?" Before I had a chance to answer his question, he was on to some other senseless topic. As bad as the encephalopathy was, it helped in situations such as that one.

As the time slowly passed I was reminded of the movie *Ground Hog Day* when the same 24 hours was repeated over and over and over again. Amy and I would spend day after day at the hospital and every evening at the marina bar. That's what my life was like. Nothing was different, and everything was the same, except for Michael who was becoming more debilitated both physically and mentally. I often wondered if he'd ever be the man I had fallen in love with. I never gave up hope, though I did wonder.

One minute Michael would seem better, the next he'd be batty and flat on his back. It was hard to watch. That happened on the day we were due to take him home from the hospital. He was improving and the encephalopathy was being held at bay. The morning Amy and I went to pick him up, the nurses had him tied to a chair, sitting on an alarm pad with his hospital tray pulled up to his chest. His eyes were bulging out of their sockets and his hair was sticking up wildly all over his head. He looked like a mad scientist. Then he started vomiting and I knew for sure he wouldn't be going home. He was still too ill.

Big Dog came into the room and agreed; we didn't go anywhere that day. I guess I knew Michael couldn't go on and on the way he was. The latest stint at Sarasota Memorial had lasted over a week with little sign of improvement. I couldn't have been more discouraged.

One monumental day Big Dog came in the hospital room for a serious conversation with us, not a chat, for he knew, too, that Michael's current health status couldn't go on as it was indefinitely. Without knowing what he was going to say, I knew by his disposition it would be hard to hear. I was glad that Michael wasn't very lucid that particular morning. While standing over the bed the doctor informed us, in a very grim voice, that Michael's meld score had gotten considerably higher than the week before, how very sick he was, and that he was in grave danger of losing his life. The doctor continued to say that a liver transplant would be the only way to save him. I don't remember what else was said, as that was enough for me to digest. The doctor left and I stood there stunned once again, looking at my husband. Should I have expected such a dire report? I didn't! My denial mechanism had been so strong that I actually felt blindsided. I had just been given an honest dose of reality. "What now?" I silently asked myself.

I thought he had been dozing when Michael looked up at me from his hospital bed, asking in the weakest of childlike voices, "Am I going to die?" My heart was breaking as I held his face in my hands and lied, "No, no, no, you are going to be fine." When he finally drifted off to sleep my emotions could no longer be hidden while memories of the past came flooding back. My entire being ached for the man who had been the love of my life and the pillar of our family for more than 30 years. Thoughts of losing him crept into my mind along with images of living my life alone. It angered and terrified me all at the same time, but mostly it saddened me. I stared through a blur of tears at my husband's gaunt face and frail body picturing him as he had once been; so handsome and so strong both physically and mentally. Feeling pure anguish, I grieved for the happiness we once had shared together as I allowed myself to wallow in self-pity.

What was wrong with me? How could I not fight for Michael? He was deteriorating before my eyes while I looked on, helplessly hoping. Was I really that incapable? Was I really going to just let him die? My thinking was slowly evolving into soul-searching. It was at that moment I realized that living in the safe state of denial that had been my existence from the time my husband became ill was no longer a choice. I needed to be more than a good caregiver; I needed to be his advocate. I needed to find that tenacious, brave girl that lived inside of me. I needed to do whatever it took to save his life. Now more than ever I had to keep my faith and find hope. I prayed to God for the courage and strength I would surely require for what I was about to undertake. As I contemplated my insurmountable mission, determination surged through me in spite of the great trepidation and fear I was feeling. Even though I didn't know where to start, I knew in my heart there had to be someone, somewhere who could help Michael. Thus began my search for a *possible miracle.*

But the questions remained: How? Where? Who?

Chapter 17

DIDN'T THEY UNDERSTAND?

September 2012

When I get bad news my first reaction is disbelief and, of course, denial, as in "there must be a mistake." That time I knew in my gut there was no mistake and that denial was not an option. But I did need clarification, so I walked up to Big Dog who was busily typing out a report at the desk. I wanted to know what all his medical jargon really meant. The doctor had been straightforward in front of Michael, but when alone with me he was brutally honest, holding nothing back and did not attempt to spare me any suffering. He delivered yet another fact to me; Michael had, at the most, three months left to live unless he received a liver transplant. The word transplant wasn't a shock anymore, but the three-month timeline was. I just stood in front of him, somberly taking in the information. As further evidence, he had me look at his computer, as he pulled up a scale of meld scores from Mayo Clinic. Looking at the scores, I saw where Michael was on their chart. It confirmed what the doctor had just recited. According to the scale I saw, my husband had three months left to live. He made a point of telling me that I needed to consider hospice for him. Hospice! "That's who is called when a patient is dying,"

I thought. The impact of his words hit me like a ton of bricks. What he had laid before me was the bare naked truth. Refusing to acknowledge the validity of what the doctor was telling me was no longer an option. Thankfully, his candid assessment forced me to embark on the process that would eventually save Michael's life.

As I walked away from him, I overheard two insensitive nurses commenting on my husband. They were saying that the hospital wasn't a holding area for someone dying of liver disease. I understood perfectly what they were talking about, but even so it was painful to hear. I wanted to tell them to be quiet, however I knew they didn't realize that I was his wife. They must all have known what I had just learned. Michael was indeed dying.

I went to the family waiting room and allowed myself some time to absorb everything I had just been told. Shouldn't I have expected this? After all, it was not the first time someone had mentioned a transplant to me. I needed to accept the reality of Michael having a liver transplant if and when he could get one. Well, sitting there crying was not going to do any good for him or for me, that was for sure. I pulled myself together and called Jack. Can you imagine? I still held on to the tiniest belief that maybe there was an off chance he wouldn't agree with what I had just been told. Jack had been keeping up with Michael's case through the Sarasota doctors. However, he was still more than surprised when I told him the latest meld score. He called the hospital immediately and talked to Big Dog, who gave him an even more thorough accounting than I had received, after which Jack called me back confirming the diagnosis. Michael's meld score was too high and rising too fast. He needed a new liver or he would surely die soon.

My whole attitude about a liver transplant had changed in a matter of minutes when I finally believed that my husband had, at the most, three months left to live. I had come full circle, wanting it for Michael, for us, more than anything in the world. Jack explained the course of action that needed to be taken. We would first apply to Mayo Clinic's transplant team as quickly as possible. He reiterated to me that Michael's chances of getting on their list was not good, but he was going to try again anyway and would present his case for the second time to the liver transplant committee the following afternoon. That was our best hope. Even though they had refused him once I was very hopeful. There were several doctors on the committee who knew of Michael's liver disease and were advocating for him. Surely they would put him on their list, as we had been patients of the Mayo Clinic for a very long time.

The next day was endless as I waited for Jack to call and give me some good news, news that only a short while ago I would have rejected. The call came late in the late afternoon, devastating me. The answer was a definite no. The Mayo transplant committee would not consider Michael for their program until he was cancer free for five years. Age had also become a factor; he would be 70 soon, which made him a high risk for transplant. That was the Clinic's protocol: no exceptions. What in the world? How could that be? Didn't they understand that his cancer had been the aggressive kind and it was three and a half years with no reoccurrence? Didn't they understand that it was their surgeon who had told me if it didn't come back in two years he had a good chance of surviving it? Didn't they understand how relative age can be? Didn't they understand that Michael was a really good man and deserved a chance to live? Didn't they understand how much his family loved him? Didn't they understand how much I loved him? Didn't they understand?

Chapter 18

THE SEARCH
Late September – Early October 2012

I t was jarring for me to acknowledge that the one hospital I had put all my confidence and trust in had turned Michael down based on their terms of acceptance for transplant recipients. Knowing how sick he was, I had been sure that Mayo would welcome him into their program immediately, especially because they had worked so arduously to save his life once already. I felt disheartened that he didn't fall within Mayo Clinic's protocol. Jack had pleaded Michael's case in front of the committee and was just as disappointed and frustrated with the ruling as I was. He told me that it was likely other hospitals would follow the same standards.

Everything was happening so fast that I didn't know what to do next and I clearly wasn't thinking things through. I hadn't wanted to consider that we may have to find another transplant center. The whole transplant process left me feeling unprepared. It was daunting for me. Knowing I desperately needed help I called Jack again and pleaded, "Help me, Jack! What should I do?" I knew he would be there for us and wasn't surprised when he answered, "I will call whoever I know at different hospitals around the country that do liver transplants and see if we can get Michael considered for their lists." His words were somewhat reassuring as Jack, being a top liver doc at Mayo Clinic, knew lots of liver docs all over. He was going to begin with Henry Ford Hospital, Northwestern University Hospital and a few other transplant centers where he knew staff. He added, "You call whoever you know that might have a connection at a transplant center. Start contacting hospitals on your own too." His words, when I think of them now, sounded kind of desperate, but they gave me conviction and spurred me on, even though I was completely overwhelmed. I didn't know where to start, but I knew I had to do what I could to rescue Michael from the merciless illness that was wreaking havoc on his body and mind. I vowed that he would not see my fear, that I would be strong and do whatever I needed to do. Although he was aware of what was happening, I found that he was somewhat removed from it at the same time given his mental status. He did not realize the gravity of his situation.

With Amy there to help with her dad, I was able to start investigating the dilemma that I faced. My first contact was with Isaac and Aida. The two of them said they would make calls to transplant facilities they knew in Florida, starting with Tampa General Hospital and the University of Miami Hospital. They were the most optimistic about Tampa. I thought it would be great if Michael could get accepted there because it was close by. I even had the idea of having him transferred right from Sarasota Memorial to Tampa General by ambulance, where he could wait for a transplant. Now that I understand how the system works, I must have been dreaming to think that might have taken place. My plan was not realistic. That is not how the transplant process works.

After sending out the word that my husband needed a transplant, I found that everyone seemed to know someone who might be able to help. I started receiving calls nonstop from family and friends with names and numbers of doctors and hospitals for me to contact. After two days of continuous phone calls, signing papers and faxing records here and there to different transplant centers, the amount of paperwork was piling up at a rate I could no longer manage. It was a gigantic undertaking at a time when I also needed to be there for my husband, who was still far from ready to leave the hospital. I called our son Adam, who was an attorney and had great organizational skills. Without hesitation he told me to have everyone call him. He would handle it. And boy did he ever!

Within days Adam became well versed in the world of liver transplantation. He first contacted Jack, who gave him a list of some of the top hospitals that did liver transplants, with instructions to call all of them. He would, in turn, continue to place calls to colleagues that he thought could help. We had no idea that there were so many transplant centers in the country. In addition, he put Adam in touch with his personal secretary who had access to 300 pages of Michael's medical records. So began the endless search!

Once unleashed, Adam went after a transplant for Michael with a vengeance. Starting with Jack's list, he got busy. If there was a hospital even remotely interested, he would send them a brief summary of Michael's case. When a facility requested more information, he would call Jack's secretary and she would forward the voluminous medical history to them. Eventually the paperwork got to be too much for her, so Adam then made his own copy of the records at his office. Every one that he contacted had a different way they wanted the file sent and received. Some centers would want part of the records, others would want only certain test results, and still others would want the whole 300 pages. At times he would have to run his fax machine all night at his office because a hospital wanted it faxed. Others would insist it be copied and sent by snail mail. It was undoubtedly exasperating for him.

Adam also contacted Michael's doctor in Sarasota for more help while still working on Jack's list. Isaac and Aida had their own group of hospitals and doctors that they were familiar with. Together Adam and Aida worked tirelessly on those connections. She was truly invaluable in the search for a transplant center that would consider Michael's plight.

In the meantime, Adam continued getting calls and referrals from many of our family members and friends. He followed up on every one of them even though he knew that most would go nowhere, as some of them were extremely bizarre. Someone even recommended an off-the-wall website where organs were traded in some fashion. I wasn't sure how that worked and didn't want to know. I didn't feel we had exhausted all other possibilities or that we were that desperate yet. Regardless, it was so heartwarming that everyone had a desire to help, even people we didn't know.

Being proactive was the only choice, so I conjured up some ideas of my own. I had become ambivalent about the means and was more focused on saving Michael. After some research I found out that living donors were an option. I would gladly give up part of my liver. What about testing me for a match as a live donor? Out of the question. I was too small; hence my liver would be too small and wouldn't be suitable for Michael's large frame. Maybe one of our kids? Amy was an exact blood type match and wanted to be a donor. I wasn't sure I wanted to go there. Nevertheless, that was out of the question too. His liver was so diseased that he needed a whole one, so a live donor would not work at all. What about Europe, Mexico or somewhere else out of the country where the protocols were different? We would go anywhere. Jack said no. None of those options was viable for Michael for various reasons and he wasn't strong enough to make the trip anyway.

While the search continued, Michael slowly regained whatever strength he could muster. When he was about ready to be released from Sarasota Memorial, a social worker presented herself to me with the suggestion that my spouse be put in a rehabilitation facility. That sounded like shades of a nursing home. "No way!" I told her, remembering my vow to Michael. She felt he'd be in danger going back to the boat, which was exactly where he would be going as I couldn't take him to the beach condo where there was a chance of him having to go back to the terrible hospital I'd had to transport him from. It would've been best if I found an acceptable place for us to rent nearby, but I hadn't had the time to pursue that option. In any case, the woman became argumentative, something I couldn't deal with just then. I called in Amy to handle her as she was also a social worker, and knew how to deal with a difficult situation like the one I was facing. After much posturing it was finally agreed upon that Michael would have physical therapy while in the hospital and it would continue at home along with home health care, which would entail a nurse and physical therapist coming to the boat to check on him daily. I could live with that. There would be no hospice or nursing home for my husband!

After more than another week at Sarasota Memorial Hospital, it was eventually time for Michael to go home. We had a welcome surprise when Amy's husband brought our oldest two grandsons for a visit. It really helped our state of mind, albeit temporary. Due to Michael's continued deterioration, our kids had decided to rotate their visits, knowing how hard it was for me to be without help. Michael literally could not be left unattended. Amy and her family went home that Sunday. Darren, our youngest son, would be the next to arrive.

During that period we found out that most of the hospitals Adam and Jack sought out had many of the same constraints as Mayo Clinic regarding liver transplantation, and after reading Michael's medical history they weren't interested. Prudently, Adam chose not to reveal how many of them merely said no without any review whatsoever. When we asked about his transplant center inquiries he came up with elaborate stories as to why he hadn't gotten an answer from them: stories that we totally believed and stories that were totally untrue. In doing so he kept our hopes alive. He was intuitive enough to know how disheartening bad news of any kind would be for us.

Our best bet after Mayo Clinic had refused Michael was Henry Ford Hospital in Detroit. Not only did Jack know the head of their transplant department, but we also had friends who knew people on the board of directors at the hospital. In fact, our son Tony was doing business with one of the transplant team doctors and thought that he might be of some assistance. Thus, a lot of calls were placed to that transplant center on Michael's behalf. We were very hopeful Henry Ford would be the one to accept him and especially wanted it to be, as our children and most of our extended family lived in the Detroit 'burbs. It was a big disappointment when they wouldn't so much as consider Michael as a potential transplant patient. Apparently rules were rules and not to be broken under any circumstances.

When we got a call from Tampa General Hospital, we thought our prayers had been answered. They had received Michael's records from Isaac's office and wanted to see him right away. I felt it was an excellent sign and undoubtedly good news. We had a car service take us for the hour and a half drive to Tampa that week. After filling out their paperwork, we were seen by a member of the hospital's transplant staff. As opposed to our interview at Mayo Clinic, we were ready to sell Michael as a great candidate for transplant. We would show them that he had a life worth saving. He wasn't bad that day and he was ready for the challenge. However, we never got the chance. Almost immediately the very congenial surgeon told us that Michael was unacceptable for transplant at Tampa General Hospital because he wasn't cancer free for five years. I was shocked! Why had they wanted to see him? Neither of us could hide our disappointment. Not wanting to give up, I asked him if my husband could be put on the list after the five year deadline was up, refusing to entertain the thought that he wouldn't be around in another year and a half. The doctor then informed us that there was another guideline that precluded anyone 70 or over from having a transplant at their facility. Since Michael would be 70 by the time he was cancer free for five years there was no way he would be accepted at Tampa General. "What the hell did we come here for?" I asked myself. I argued with the physician that some 50-year-olds weren't as young as my husband and didn't have the great lifestyle he had. The doctor agreed, but said there was nothing he could do. He sat on the exam table throughout the entire 15 minutes that we had been allotted while Michael sat on a chair. He had not so much as touched my husband the whole time; he only talked to him. It was a total waste of our emotions and energy.

Even though he wasn't himself, Michael knew enough to feel defeated. I tried to remain positive on our way home and the rest of the week, but it did little to lift his spirits as calls were coming in on a daily basis with negative responses. The episode at Tampa General was a real blow. Luckily Adam was not discouraged. He had contacted so many hospitals that even he lost track of the number of them. During that time I never gave up hope and Adam never stopped trying.

During our search, our very good friend, Rabbi Harold Loss, told us about one of his friends in Michigan, who had a lung transplant at Cleveland Clinic. Apparently his buddy knew one of the members on the lung transplant team quite well. We all thought this was something we should definitely pursue. Yet when we heard the name of the individual we were initially flummoxed as to how to handle it. Michael had been involved in an altercation with Harold's friend, Michael Roth, years ago over our kids and they hadn't spoken since. How could we call him for a favor, a gigantic one at that? Well, who cared? We needed help sooner rather than later! Harold, along with another friend who was also close to Michael Roth, convinced us that we should make contact with him, as they had laid the groundwork for Michael and I and were sure he would be willing to do whatever he could to assist us. In any case, what was the point of standing on principle when fighting for your life?

Having his meds adjusted once again, Michael's mind was a bit clearer than it had been and he was able to have a simple conversation, so it was decided he would be the one to make the initial call. The past being an unwanted memory for Harold's friend, Michael, as well as for us, he was more than happy to help. With a somewhat hopeful feeling, we turned the good connection over to Adam, who got in touch with him immediately and I mean that same day. As luck would have it, our new acquaintance was on his way to Cleveland when Adam called. He and his wife would be attending a party for the lung transplant department that very night. He said he would speak with Dr. Marie Budev, Medical Director of Cleveland Clinic's Lung Transplant Program, on Michael's behalf. That's about all he could do; the rest would be up to her. We had hopes that she would contact the director of the liver transplant department, but there was no way to know for sure. Although it was only an introduction, it was a big one, and it made us feel more positive than we had in a long time.

The next day Adam received a call from a liver transplant coordinator at Cleveland Clinic requesting information regarding Michael's medical history. It appeared that our prayers were indeed being answered. At Cleveland Clinic someone had immediately grasped the seriousness of my husband's liver disease and his urgent need for a liver transplant. They were going to, at the very least, look at his health records. We prayed it would go farther than that.

Adam was ready with the entire report from Mayo Clinic even though they had only asked for certain parts of the document. He reasoned that the more data he sent to the transplant team the better. That night at his office he was getting ready to start faxing the countless pages when an IT friend of his, happened to call. In no time Adam's friend took over. He had Adam send him a copy of the document. With that in hand, he set up a website with Michael's huge medical file on it. That way the hospital, once it accessed the site, merely needed to read it online or copy it themselves if need be. It saved valuable time, which we didn't have a lot of, and tons of paperwork. Because they had asked for only specific items I'm sure they were surprised when, with the help of the new website, they had obtained Michael's 300 page case history by the following morning. We were told later that they had never received a reply to their request in such a timely fashion nor with as much information, which definitely helped to facilitate their assessment.

The following day Cleveland Clinic called, asking for a PET scan and blood test to be done in Sarasota as quickly as possible, because the latest ones from Mayo Clinic were not current enough. I knew they would be looking for signs of pancreatic and liver cancer. Would the pursuit of the awful disease ever stop? Probably not! We got the order for everything that was needed from Isaac, who set up the appointments. That next day Michael went through the various testing. I had the written results along with the scan overnighted to the transplant team, as they needed the actual hard copy. In the meantime, Isaac told me the outcome of the tests were good; my husband was cancer free as far as the Sarasota radiologists could determine. My jitters were palpable as we waited to hear back from the transplant coordinator in Cleveland.

At the very same time that Cleveland Clinic was looking into Michael's case, Adam got a response from Northwestern University Hospital in Illinois. He wisely didn't tell me about their request for information because he realized I was more than overwhelmed with all that was happening with Cleveland Clinic. Northwestern wanted Michael's medical file and was prepared to at least assess him for their transplant program, regardless of the fact he was not cancer free for five years or that he was almost 70. Jack's relationship with a doctor there seemed to have paid off.

As Adam navigated his way through the liver transplantation community, he had found out how to get things accomplished. His goal was to do whatever it took to save Michael's life. Months later I found out that, with help, he had applied to well over 20 hospitals, all of which had said no. Mayo Clinic, Henry Ford and Tampa General were the only ones that had given us reason to hope and in the end they had all refused Michael. There was Northwestern Hospital, but we didn't know what they would say and they were taking too much time; time we didn't have. Our hope was reborn with Cleveland Clinic.

The wait continued! On Friday of that week I got the call we were praying for. The liver transplant team wanted to see Michael at Cleveland Clinic on the following Monday to do an evaluation. Was it really happening? I had waited for a positive response, but I was shaken up by the call just the same. The transplant coordinator forewarned me that Michael would endure a thorough vetting process during the upcoming week. There would be innumerable tests, ultrasounds, scans, examinations and interviews of all kinds. I felt terrible putting him through all that given how very weak and ill he was, but there was no alternative. It would undoubtedly be miserable for him. At the end of that time the transplant committee would likely get together to decide whether they would put him on their list. The thoughts of my husband having a liver transplant were becoming a possible reality.

Earlier in the week, Darren had come to spend time with us, giving me some much needed support. He made arrangements for us to fly to Cleveland on Sunday together. Going it alone with Michael was out of the question. I didn't know how encephalopathic he would be from one minute to the next and his walking ability was always questionable. We were grateful to have Darren's help. I prepared for the trip while he took care of everything else, including Michael. Thank goodness he was there.

The day before we left for Cleveland was our wedding anniversary. With what lay ahead of us, I really wasn't in the mood to party, but Michael wanted to celebrate, our kids wanted us to celebrate, and our friends at the marina restaurant wanted us to celebrate, so I was outnumbered. When we got to the restaurant that night, there were flowers and a beautiful cake waiting. With Darren and our friends we were able to enjoy our anniversary that would have otherwise been melancholy. When the musician played a special song for us, Mickey asked me to dance. It was so very difficult to hold in my emotions. I knew it took all of his strength to stand, let alone walk or even dance. As he held me in his arms I felt that dance was for me and for a moment in time I let all thoughts of the uncertain future go.

Packing for a few days was the easy part. Getting Michael to Tampa, on the plane to Cleveland, and to the hotel was the hard part. Darren and I were hoping he would be good enough to fly when it was time to go and by chance he was, though only slightly. Darren had rented a car and drove us to Tampa. That's when my daffy husband insisted the car be filled up at the airport gas station. I didn't think there was one there and given that his mind was not all there, I told our son not to take his advice, but he was so insistent that Darren gave in, following his directions. Big mistake! What were we thinking listening to him? Of course, there wasn't a gas station in sight and it cost a fortune to turn the car in on empty. Oh well! Once at the airport Darren was so frustrated he chose to take over, even though Michael tried to interfere. As if he was talking to one of his kids, Darren told Michael to sit down in the wheelchair he had secured for him and wait with me. Thankfully Mickey gave in and sat quietly in the chair. It was as if the roles were reversed and Michael was the son. Soon we were off to Cleveland without a problem.

Chapter 19

FOR OR AGAINST

October 2012

Once we arrived in Cleveland safely, Darren went home to his family. For the sake of convenience we stayed at a hotel that was attached to the Clinic. Adam arrived early the next morning to help us with the grueling week of examinations that lay ahead. The first meeting was with our new transplant coordinator. We had been turned over to her by the initial coordinator who was with us during the application process. Our new one would help Michael and me maneuver through the next days of endless exams, tests and interviews. Upon meeting with her, she explained what we were to expect in the week to come. The last few months had left me dazed and on autopilot. Knowing we were actually at Cleveland Clinic in hopes of getting put on their liver transplant list caused me to wake up. This was getting damn serious!

Our next appointment was with a liver transplant surgeon, Dr. Cristiano Quintini. As we approached the meeting, the three of us felt as if we were going to be on stage. We had to be perfect, as a good impression was imperative. My husband needed to be seen as a deserving transplant recipient. I call it a meeting because Michael was not examined. It was the same as the appointment with the doctor at Tampa General and Mayo Clinic; we merely talked. Cristiano explained to us that the committee's major concern was the possibility of recurring pancreatic cancer. Liver cancer was not mentioned. It was expected there would be ample concern over cancer. We were told that if Michael were to be accepted into their program and a liver were to become available for him, they would do exploratory surgery prior to the transplant. It would be the last way to make sure that he was cancer free. If cancerous lesions were to be found, he would be closed up and the organ he was to get would be given to another patient who was prepped and ready to go in a nearby pre-op room. That was not the best news. Knowing they would be looking for cancer so closely made me feel sick to my stomach. As the appointment continued, Michael's personality won over the intelligent surgeon in a heartbeat. Before we left the office Cristiano said to him, "I'm going to get you a new liver and you are going to live forever." That was better news! I fell in love with the cocky doctor immediately, for he had shown us a light at the end of the very dark tunnel we were currently in. I hoped the whole transplant staff was that confident. More and more I was thinking that a transplant could happen, although as usual, the cancer business caused me great misgivings.

With Adam by my side we watched as my poor man went through hell during that week of testing, poking and prodding. I couldn't count how many times his blood was taken and at that point in his liver disease, he was no simple stick. He would come out of the lab time after time with bandages up and down his skinny bruised arms. The transplant doctors ordered copious tests: from scans to ultra sounds, from MRIs to X-rays, from endoscopy to colonoscopy, to pulmonary tests. He was seen by numerous specialists: from an endocrinologist, to a dermatologist, to a urologist, to a cardiologist, to a gastroenterologist/hepatologist, to an oncologist, to a radiologist, to a pulmonologist and more. These different docs added their own particular tests too.

Many of them were searching for cancer anywhere in or on his body where it might be lurking.

There were appointments with a psychiatrist, a social worker, a dietician and many with our transplant coordinator. They all wanted to know about the quality of Michael's life and if it was one worth saving. It appeared that no stone would be left unturned. It made me uneasy and apprehensive the whole time.

When the infectious disease doc got hold of Michael he was given a slew of injections and vaccinations. He would need all of them if he was selected for transplant.

The cardiologist ordered a stress test for Michael, as they needed to know if he could physically withstand the surgery, given his weakened state. That hadn't occurred to me and made me worry it was possible that he wasn't strong enough for a liver transplant. I wondered how they were going to do a stress test when there was no way that he could walk on a treadmill or go on a bicycle for that matter. There was a solution for everything. They simply induced stress through medication given by IV while he lay on a table. Mickey seemed to take it all in stride.

During Michael's appointment with the pulmonologist, it was noted that he had an excessive buildup of fluid in his lungs. The doctor wanted it aspirated and analyzed. I was told that there was a potential that cancer cells were in the fluid. When he was having trouble breathing at Sarasota Memorial, the doctors had discovered the fluid, but no one had ever mentioned the word cancer in reference to it. Michael would never get a transplant if that were the case. However, since the procedure to remove it was invasive, the transplant team felt that in his sickly physical state the danger of the aspiration causing infection was far too great and he was also still at risk of getting pneumonia, so they didn't want to take a chance. It was decided to put it on the back burner temporarily and watch his lungs closely. I thought to myself, "Is there anything else you'd like to frighten me with?" You'd think that I would be numb to all the shocks I had to endure regarding Michael's health, but they still sent me into a tailspin.

As the appointments continued some were more memorable than others. The gastroenterologist/hepatologist was one of our main docs, as he dealt with the liver. We really liked the soft-spoken man, who had at one time worked with Jack at Mayo Clinic. He seemed positive about Michael's chances for getting a transplant. He surprised me when he added that we would be expected to relocate in Cleveland if the transplant committee accepted my husband at the end of the week. With an even voice I told him, "We'll stay if that's what we need to do." The doctor wanted us to be clear about the gravity of the situation, so he then added that Michael now had about two months left of his life and he surely wouldn't make it if he went home.

As for my guy, the encephalopathy evidently helped to tune out that part of the conversation, as he never mentioned it to me. The only thing he seemed to focus on was that we were going to have to spend time in Cleveland. Can you imagine that after the meeting, Mickey told me he had no intention of staying in Cleveland past Friday? Right, like I was going to give him a say in it! Not a chance!

That appointment put me in a state of profound depression. I didn't want to accept that my husband had weeks left to live. No one, not Michael or anyone else knew how I felt. For them I kept my positive Pollyanna attitude, but unwanted thoughts invaded my nights as I became more and more inundated with thoughts of the surgery, recovery, all the meds and how absolutely wretched all of it would be. The worse thought of all was Michael dying. Leaving Cleveland without out my husband, going on our boat by myself and having to live alone kept me awake at night. My sleep was being sacrificed to the fear of the future. How could I handle it all? Attempts to relax and clear my mind were futile. I pictured the stop sign that my PTSD therapist had recommended to me and it did help somewhat.

During the days we were busy nonstop, which was the best antidote for my nerves. Most of the appointments scheduled were with the doctors and staff who were members of the all-important liver transplant committee. They would be the ones to decide if Michael met their criteria for a transplant. Adam and I would confer after each appointment as to whether they were "for or against" him getting a new liver. Up to the point when we saw the oncologist we thought most were "for". We knew that cancer could be our one major roadblock, so the consultation with and the conclusions of the oncologist were of great significance.

Once again there was no examination. The oncologist asked a lot of questions, taking notes while I spoke. His job after meeting with us, was to collect data from studies on survival rates of pancreatic cancer patients whose case histories were similar to that of Michael's, as far as the stage of cancer, the size of the tumor, where it was located, the treatment that followed and the length of time he had been cancer free. The doctor would then present his findings to the committee when they had their weekly meeting. The physician seemed extremely knowledgeable in his field, which made me all the more nervous because his questions were very detailed and to the point. It almost seemed as though he was trying to find a reason for Michael not to have the transplant. When Adam and I looked at each other after that appointment we knew without speaking what the other was thinking, simultaneously mouthing the word "against". Thankfully, I don't think Michael understood how bad we felt about that particular appointment.

As strange as it sounds, the most positive appointment was with the doc who did the colonoscopy. Standing over Michael in recovery, he told us that he had also worked with Jack at Mayo Clinic and he was the head of the powerful committee that would make the decision as to Michael's eligibility for transplant. I could tell that he really took to my hubby. He felt neither the pancreatic cancer nor his age were problematic. Therefore, the consensus was that he was a definite "for". Even with the encephalopathy, all the doctors seemed to get Michael's personality. They liked him and that was very advantageous.

Toward the end of the week we had two seemingly effortless appointments, one with a social worker and one with a dietician, both liver transplant specialists. The night before we were to meet with the social worker, Michael called Amy for tips on how to handle the interview and what to wear. It was curious that meeting made him more jumpy than all the others. "Be yourself," was our daughter's advice. Because of the encephalopathy that was somewhat difficult, as Michael was never himself anymore.

At the social worker's office, Michael sat between Adam and me, leaning forward, elbows on knees, very hyper and very animated. The social worker, Cassie Rosenbaum, inputted on her computer the answers to all questions she asked. Being a liver transplant candidate, the question of alcohol use was bound to come up. Neither Adam nor I thought there was a need to coach Michael on how he should answer the simple question. He only needed to be honest. Were we ever mistaken! When she asked the question, "Do you drink alcohol?" the reply was immediate. Without hesitation Michael answered, "I have always loved to pound down scotch. Every day I used to come home from work and have a few." What the hell was he talking about? He sounded like an alcoholic! That's just the kind of person who would have a problem getting a new liver. Not only was it way too much information, it wasn't even close to the truth. Adam and I sat upright and quickly looked at each other behind Michael's back. He was then asking the question, "How much liquor will I be able to drink after the transplant? What about beer and . . ." Before any more damage could be done Adam loudly interrupted. "Listen to me, I lived with Michael throughout most of my life and never saw him pound down scotch, let alone even drink scotch and if he did drink, it was not at home. When we would go out he would sometimes have vodka." I immediately concurred. The sheepish look on Michael's face told us that he knew he had made a colossal mistake. In the meantime, Cassie never stopped typing. Yikes!

I left the office deflated and shook up, thinking we had just added an "against" to our list. On the other hand, Adam was furious. He told Michael in his lawyerly voice, "Only answer the question asked and with short answers." Michael now thought he had ruined his chance of getting a transplant. We knew the social worker was part of the committee and her interview had been very important. Pouting like a naughty child, he begged me to go back to her office and tell her he didn't mean it. He was so upset with himself that sympathy took over. I agreed to try and see her again. I called her phone number and when she heard the urgency in my voice she had me come back to her office right away. Sitting with Cassie once again, but alone this time, I told her what Michael had been like before he got sick. Of course, I added how he should have answered her question on the topic of alcohol. It was her profession to read people and she had read Michael correctly from the beginning, understanding that he was encephalopathic. Her report would not say that he was an excessive drinker, only a social one. She commented to me how young he seemed and how much fun he appeared to be. Cassie liked him. What had been a for sure "against" had turned into a "for". She informed me that if Michael was accepted into the liver transplant program she would be our social worker and would be there for both of us if we needed anything at all. I left her office with the best of feelings.

Once we finished with the social work interview we headed for the dietician. I shouldn't have been surprised when the same thing that happened with Cassie happened again with the dietician. Michael started mentioning Kentucky Fried Chicken and McDonald's. He wanted to know that he could eat that junk food after the transplant. Adam and I couldn't believe what he was talking about. It was important for her to know that after getting a new liver Michael would live a healthy lifestyle. We had to revert to damage control again during that meeting.

Just when I thought we were coming to the end of our scheduled appointments, we found out that we were required to take a class on liver transplantation. We wheeled Michael into the classroom and sat at the back of the room. He was not doing well that day, but the lecture was mandatory. He quickly fell asleep in the wheelchair and stayed that way throughout the entire class. After getting tons of information on paper, one of the instructors went over the whole process with us, from first being evaluated to being accepted, finding a match, the waiting time, and what was expected of the patient, the caregiver and the family. Then she discussed the surgery, hospital stay and recovery period while at Cleveland Clinic. She also covered all the meds and their side effects. We learned about the recuperation at home and the months and years after transplant. Furthermore, we would be assigned more transplant coordinators to help us along the way. The amount of information was intimidating. We would be expected to carry around a large notebook that included everything we had just gone over. I thought, "Give me the binder and I will thankfully carry it everywhere with me for the rest of my life!" To receive the coveted notebook meant that Michael would be listed for transplant. All of it was pending acceptance by the committee.

The agonizing week that we had been through produced some good news. The doctors and techs had been unable to find the slightest trace of cancer anywhere in or on Michael's body, and believe me, they really looked for it everywhere. By the time the appointments were over, Michael was totally exhausted, black and blue all over his body, and was in such a weakened state that he was almost constantly in a wheelchair. His sensitivity to cold had increased, making it unbearable to be in the hotel room with him, where he had the temperature set at no lower than 75 F. One evening, Adam and I were sitting in the room with Michael, sweating profusely. Upon reaching his limit, Adam took off his shirt and eventually had to leave our room. When Mickey fell asleep and I couldn't take it either, I joined our son across the hall, where he had the air conditioning in his room turned on full blast even though it was freezing outside. If I hadn't had to keep an eye on Michael I would have spent the night there. The problem we had with regulating the heat was ongoing. My honey always believed I had the temperature set well below where it was appropriate.

After three and a half days Adam left to go home. The tension increased as Friday approached. Michael's fate could be decided on that day. All thoughts were focused on the transplant committee's verdict: "for" or "against" and there was no way to tell.

Chapter 20

THE VERDICT
Mid-October 2012

It was really strange. For months I wouldn't contemplate a liver transplant for Michael but suddenly I was praying for it. I felt anguish at the possibility that he might not be accepted into the transplant program at Cleveland Clinic and at the same time I was distressed about all that lay ahead of us if he were. The whole subject was so very hard to imagine.

With the end of our first week in sight, we had another meeting with our transplant coordinator. She gave us no indication as to how Michael's appointments had gone or in what direction the committee might lean. What she did tell us was that the determination as to whether or not Michael would be chosen for the liver transplant list would definitely occur on that Friday afternoon. It was a huge step forward. Through all the applications to all the hospitals and through all the tests, we had wanted to get to that point. My safe state of denial was long gone.

Our coordinator told me to keep my phone handy on Friday from mid to late afternoon. That's when she would call with the committee's decision. She stated that if accepted, the transplant team expected us to stay in Cleveland until a donor liver became available and for at least two months afterwards while Michael recovered. I was prepared for the first part, but what I didn't know was that we would be required to stay in Cleveland for a very long time after the surgery. It didn't matter, because by then I was perfectly fine with the prospect of living there, not really caring how long it might be, as long as I could take my husband home with me when I left.

I also found out that another week of appointments had been scheduled for Michael. Some of the previous test results had shown possible problems unrelated to cancer, and therefore most likely due to his liver disease. However, no matter what the cause, these issues needed to be addressed whether the committee accepted him or not.

Our plan was to stay in Cleveland at least another week and, optimistically, more. I decided it would be more comfortable and affordable for us if we moved to a hotel on the property that had more suitable accommodations: a separate bedroom, a small living room and a kitchenette. On Friday morning we made the transition to the new hotel. I was certainly trying to think positive. That kept us busy for a while. Michael was alert and, to a degree, aware of the finding that was going to be made about him later that day, so we were able to share feelings, which made the passing hours more bearable for me. Our kids arrived in Cleveland to be with us when we received the expected call. They were as anxious as we were and knew we needed their company no matter what the verdict was, especially if Michael was turned down.

Unbeknownst to me, while we were in Cleveland, Adam was still communicating with the Northwestern Hospital Transplant Center. They had finally decided to evaluate Michael for their program. I was so involved with Cleveland Clinic at that time that I had no thoughts of other hospitals. What I found out later was, that our kids were there not only to support us, but had plans, if Michael was not accepted at Cleveland, to whisk us off to Chicago, where there was an appointment set up for him at Northwestern Hospital the following week.

Once everyone arrived at our hotel, we spent the afternoon speculating as to how the appointments had gone and which of the doctors and staff would be advocates for Michael, trying to tally up who might be "for" and who might be "against." The only good that did was occupy the time. We prayed the majority of votes would be "for." When that got old, nervous eating seemed to be the next option. Even though the call wasn't expected until later in the day, I stared at my phone that I had laid on the table in the hotel dining room, willing it to ring. The not knowing was debilitating and just plain old miserable. I was on edge the entire afternoon.

All of a sudden the phone flashed, informing me there was a message waiting. I panicked! "Why the hell didn't it ring?" I asked louder than necessary. Our server interrupted, "The phone service in the restaurant is bad." Upon examining the phone I saw there was a Cleveland area code on the screen. I froze, not able to move for a split second, then ran at top speed out of the dining room, phone in hand, with my family looking after me. I was shaking so badly that accessing my voice mail was difficult. It was our coordinator! She wanted me to call her back immediately. As I listened to her message there was no indication in her voice if Michael had been accepted or not. I called her back instantaneously, hardly being able to handle the simple chore. It felt as though the phone rang and rang and rang, and then there she was. Wasting no time, she said the words I had been praying to hear. Michael was being put on the list for a liver transplant. I was astounded! I was ecstatic!

It had been a unanimous decision by all those attending the committee meeting that my husband be a candidate for transplant pending the test results from the following week and approval from the state. It was the first I had heard about the state's involvement. She assured me there wouldn't be a problem. I couldn't talk to her just then; I was too hysterical as emotions seized me and wouldn't let go. With tears streaming down my face I ran back to the restaurant and grabbed Michael telling him and everyone else who was in shouting distance, "We are getting a new liver!" It was hardly a sure thing at that time, but I didn't care. Feeling positive felt really good for a change.

I couldn't think beyond that day and the committee's ruling. After months of agonizing over what was going to happen to my husband, there was finally more than just a direction; we had a definite course of action, with hopefully a good resolution. I wasn't going to think about all the ramifications of Michael being chosen for a liver transplant. We were all going to enjoy some good news that day and celebrate. Tomorrow would be soon enough to contemplate the future and all the unpredictability that it held for us.

Chapter 21

BRING IT ON!

Mid-October 2012

*T*here we were in Cleveland and it was the next day. I couldn't silence my mind. Fortunately the two thoughts that I avoided were that Michael wouldn't get the transplant or when he did, how very serious that type of surgery was going to be. There was no benefit in thinking about all that, so I didn't. Instead I focused on getting us organized for the months ahead. The Pollyanna girl was back! It was a new kind of denial for me. However, I did continue to marvel at the magnitude of what lay ahead, letting it engulf my entire being. My family was with me, but still the responsibility lay at my feet. It was then time to get busy.

The more I thought about what was going to happen, the less Mickey was capable of doing the same. Even though he wanted to control what was to transpire, I couldn't let that occur. He came up with an illogical plan of leasing an apartment nearby and then renting a car for me to drive. I indulged him, but I can tell you now, there was no way in hell I was leaving the security of being on Cleveland Clinic grounds and no way in hell I would be driving in the snow, which was always considerable during Cleveland winters. He was getting sicker by the day, thus being close to the hospital was imperative. To placate him, Amy drove us here and there looking at apartments that I agreed to follow up on, yet had no intention of even considering. At the same time I went ahead with my own plans, knowing as soon as he got comfy in our new efficiency he'd adjust and eventually forget about the possibility of moving elsewhere.

With my sweet daughter at my side, we set up the two small rooms where we would be residing. I confiscated dishes from the hotel restaurant, fixed up the tiny kitchenette with a couple of small appliances and filled the fridge with healthy food. I had only packed enough clothing for five days, so I purchased additional garments to keep us warm in the frigid snowy months that lay ahead, especially for Michael. Given that everything went as planned, we would be wintering in cold snowy Cleveland not warm sunny Florida. Ugh!

We finished the rest of the appointments the following week, at which time we found out that a third transplant coordinator would be assigned to us. It seemed just as we were getting used to one, there would be another to get acquainted with. We had learned that if Michael was to get a transplant, there would be even more to come. Each had his or her own area of expertise, making them all necessary to the process. Our first appointment after being placed on the transplant list was with the new coordinator who had a bevy of instructions for me. I was the one totally in charge at that point, which caused me to listen intently, taking notes when needed. Number three would be with us through the stand-by stage of the transplant process. She would be the one to place the call to us when and if a liver became available for my man. Also, if there were any health problems along the way, she was my go-to person. It was comforting to know that I had someone to call day or night if need be. Michael still wasn't officially on the list due to the awaited test results and the approval from the state, but hopefully that would come soon. Everyone said not to worry. We continued with our coordinator as if he were already listed. She even gave me the sought after notebook for transplant patients with instructions to study it cover to cover.

While we were in limbo waiting, our kids would come to keep us company. When Darren visited, he chauffeured us around Cleveland, helping me get various errands done while taking care of Michael at the same time. On one of those missions he assisted me in obtaining a new phone and service. Needing to be well connected to the Clinic at all times was compulsory. Once the test results were in and the state said yes, the call could come at any moment. During the class we had taken the week before, the instructor had been adamant about the caregiver being on call 24/7, phone charged and on his or her person at all times. We needed to be ready to go to the hospital immediately when our coordinator phoned that there was a liver available. Most transplants are not like any other planned surgeries where there is a date, time and surgeon; we wouldn't know any of that until there was a donor match. Our coordinator had informed us that Michael would be near the top of the liver transplant list because of his high meld score. In addition, he was an AB blood type and could be matched to another AB or a A, B or O. That would give him better odds. She added that because they did so many liver transplants at Cleveland Clinic in a year, the surgery could happen sooner rather than later. The bottom line was that we should be prepared for the transplant to happen at any time, thus a good phone with good reception was a necessity.

The one study I was very curious about was the analysis the oncologist had done, as thoughts of cancer continued to plague us. Even though all the many tests and scans Michael had gone through hadn't shown any traces of the dreaded disease, the same frightful feelings had been reborn again with a new intensity during the transplant assessment. It was good news when we were given the report that the cancer specialist had read to the transplant committee. It was what we had wanted to hear for a long time; Michael's chances of having recurring pancreatic cancer were unlikely. In fact, he had added, his probability of getting the disease again was about the same as anyone else sitting on that very transplant committee. We were so relieved I wanted to kiss that doctor for his diligence and optimism. Cleveland Clinic alone had taken the time to do the research based on Michael's individual case. I wanted to scream it out loud to all the transplant centers that had refused my husband a chance at life based on his cancer risk.

That week we had another meeting with Cassie, our social worker. Her report to the committee had also been very positive. We were elated with the prospect of Michael getting a transplant and couldn't help giving her a hug to show our gratitude. Her next job was giving aid to my husband, the patient, and me, the caregiver, with any emotional problems that we might encounter during our stay at Cleveland Clinic and afterwards. She went more in-depth than they had in the class, listing chronologically what we may experience. First, we would go through the comprehensive draining process of getting approved. Second, was the subsequent feeling of buoyancy once that happened. We had just finished stages one and two and we were about to enter stage three, which was waiting for the call that a donor liver was available. Cassie explained what could happen during that time. There was no way to know when the transplant would take place, thus keeping us at a high level of anticipation. It would most likely be a very tense time for both of us, especially if there were dry runs. It was possible that we would get a call that there was a donor liver and rush to the hospital. Michael would get prepped for surgery. If there were a problem with the organ or the donor, we would be sent back to the hotel and there would be no transplant that day. That didn't sound like fun, but it seemed very improbable that it would ever happen. I stashed that in the back of my mind, the one thing I didn't need was something else to contemplate.

Once called, we would be offered the liver. Offer: what an odd word to use! Cassie went on; we would get a call from our transplant coordinator who would then make an offer with a brief description of the donor, such as old or young and the type of injury or disease that caused the death and we would be told if the liver had been compromised at all. That was another thought that had never occurred to me. After that, there would be a decision to make as to whether we wanted to go ahead with the transplant. That whole part was all new to me and shook me up as well, since I would be the one to do the deciding. I stashed that away too. Fourth, there were all kinds of emotions we would experience in regards to the donor. I tried not to think of what would have to occur for Michael's life to be saved. After the transplant we'd be able to write a letter to the family through Lifebanc, the transplant network. I knew that would be hard to do and knew I would do it anyway if my husband lived. Fifth was the strain of the surgery and the stay in the hospital. It would be an extremely stressful time. Sixth was leaving Cleveland Clinic for home, which would be hard. Thoughts of getting PTSD again entered my mind. I certainly didn't need that to happen. Last was the constant connection we would have with the Cleveland Clinic transplant team for the rest of Michael's life. My head was reeling when she finished. I'm glad that throughout our period at the Clinic we were getting information in bits and pieces. If I had known at the onset the extent of what we would go through, there was no way I could have wrapped my arms around it all. However, having the transplant staff by my side every step of the way helped ease my distress.

We finally got settled in our Cleveland residence, safely on the Clinic grounds. If Michael needed medical help it was minutes away. His plans of living any-where else were forgotten. Our children all had gone home to be with their families. My sister and her husband had left on a long vacation. Everyone had gone back to his or her own lives and routines. If I needed family, our kids were only a few hours away. There was no adjusting to the new way of life.

There was only learning to live with it and getting through it. Did I feel sorry for myself? You bet I did!

Michael finished the rest of his tests and all the results came back good. Towards the end of that second week the state had said yes. He was not only near the top he was, indeed, number one in his blood type on the liver transplant list. That's how very sick he was. On Wednesday Oct. 17, the waiting officially started and so did an existence laced with fear of what lay ahead along with hope for tomorrow. From that time forward I felt as if I had been put on high alert. I was always jumpy and could hardly sleep at night.

As if our challenge with the pancreatic cancer wasn't enough in a lifetime, we were about to endure another big one. I thought many times, "Bring it on! I don't want to be stuck in this debilitating nightmare any longer."

Chapter 22

DRY RUNS
Mid to Late October 2012

With the enthusiasm and excitement we had felt when Michael was first listed in the transplant program a thing of the past, we waited as his health continued to decline. The worst part was the encephalopathy. One day he was good, the next day terrible; it was always downhill, never great. I was spending every minute with what appeared to be a very drunk husband. He was extremely cold all of the time, no matter how he was dressed. The tiredness was ever increasing and he spent a great deal of everyday in bed. The itching was so bad he would scratch himself until he bled. I took him to see the dermatologist who sent him for biweekly light therapy, which seemed to help.

The gastroenterologist/hepatologist was extremely concerned about Michael's degenerating condition. Blood tests were ongoing as a way to track his meld score amongst a zillion other things. The results showed his score to be continually on the rise. A year previously he had weighed close to 195 pounds. When he weighed in at the office he was barely 150. It pained me to see him undressed. He had bones sticking out all over his scrawny frame and looked as though he hadn't had a thing to eat in weeks. Needless to say, he was becoming weaker and weaker. I prayed he would last.

The doctor gave me his cellphone number with instructions to call or text any time in case there was a problem. If I needed anything at all, the coordinator was available day or night. Almost immediately I made friends with the hotel staff. I knew those wonderful strangers were also there for me. I especially bonded with other caregivers; we had a lot in common. It went unsaid that we were all part of a support system. That was how we lived for the time being. But, not for long!

Ten days into our waiting period, early on a Monday morning, as I was getting ready to take Mickey to the Clinic for his light treatment, the phone rang. Whenever I heard that sound during that interim period I would jump out of my skin. If it was a Cleveland area code my heart would start racing and my adrenaline would surge. That's exactly what happened that day. It was our coordinator! "We have an offer for your husband," she said calmly. I knew it could happen, but so soon? I hadn't expected it and wasn't ready! As I tried to pull myself together, she told me the liver was compromised because of the age of the donor, yet the surgeons felt it was a good match. Surely they wouldn't want to do a transplant if the organ wasn't in good shape. As long as the decision was at my discretion I told her I would call her right back with an answer. We had been advised during our class that taking a few minutes to gather thoughts and ascertain what to do was perfectly acceptable when making that life altering decision, so I took some time and called Jack. He was my safety net; I didn't have the same relationship with anyone at Cleveland Clinic as of yet. I relayed to him the information our coordinator had given me and he told me to hold on while he checked with a surgeon from the transplant team at Mayo Clinic. When he came back on the phone he told me to take the offer. Even with the go-ahead from him, I was reluctant. It was the most important judgment call I had ever made, but in the end there really wasn't anything else I could do. I called the coordinator back giving her my answer. She in turn rattled off instructions for Michael not to eat or take his meds; I was to take him to the admitting desk at the hospital immediately. I'm sure there were other things she told me, but that is all that I can recall.

Michael was in his usual mentally unbalanced state, so getting him ready to go was not an easy chore. He was more than agitated about not eating breakfast. The ride on the shuttle to the hospital seemed to take an eternity. Finally, at 9 a.m., we were checked in and taken to the transplant floor. Once in the room it was non-stop activity. There was an EKG, an X-ray, blood to be drawn and IVs to be hooked up, among other tests that needed to be completed before surgery. The surgeon came by to check on Michael, making sure that the liver would be the right size for him. That was another thought that hadn't occurred to me. Of course it made sense that size would matter. I remembered being told that I was too small to be a living donor for Michael when I thought that might be an option.

By 11 a.m., he was prepped and ready. At first, every couple of hours our coordinator would call my cellphone with an update. I couldn't believe it was taking so long. As the day wore on, the updates were coming further and further apart while Michael was getting more and more hungry by the moment and getting more and more encephalopathic from having not taken his meds. The coordinator had said it would take some time, but it was hard to have patience.

I reached our family, telling them to come to Cleveland. Today was the day. I had been told the donor was from out of state and I would get a call letting me know once the surgery had started to procure the liver. That would give family plenty of time to drive the three hours to the Clinic. Michael wanted to see them before he was taken to surgery. Amy arrived first and the waiting continued. The last call from our coordinator came around 9 p.m., a good 12 hours after we had arrived at the hospital. Placidly she told me, "The liver isn't good and the transplant is not going to happen today." It was a huge disappointment. By 10 p.m., Michael, Amy and I were back at the hotel and the rest of the family had turned around to go home. So, that was what a dry run was all about. I thought we had been prepared for everything, but even though I knew it was a possibility, we weren't prepared for it to happen. I hated it!

The next morning Michael was a complete wreck from not taking his medications the day before. I took him for his light treatment anyway. Also, I felt he should see his doctor after what he had been through and because of how sick he seemed to be that day. We met with our coordinator, only talking to her briefly. She would set up an appointment for him to see the gastroenterologist/hepatologist that afternoon.

There was no time to go back to the hotel for lunch, so we chose the cafeteria at the Clinic for ease. Amy was helping Michael manage through the soup line, who after the difficult day before was experiencing a moderate amount of confusion over his choice of soup. Suddenly my phone rang. I saw the Cleveland area code, but was not flustered by it that time. After all, we had just left the transplant department. It was our coordinator, who I assumed was calling in regards to our afternoon appointment. She asked me where we were and I told her we were about to have lunch. "Don't let Michael eat!" she practically screamed into the phone. "We have another offer for your husband." No way! I couldn't believe it! The timing was insane! She told me about the liver and the donor. Another one that was compromised, because of something to do with the bile ducts. "Was there ever a perfect liver?" I asked. "Rarely," she answered. However, the donor was young and the liver itself was in good shape. It sounded better than yesterday's offer; but the bile duct issue sounded ominous to me. Once more I needed some time to think it over and, of course, call my buddy.

First, I flew into the restaurant to get Michael before he downed his soup. He definitely was not a happy camper leaving it behind. In fact, he was more concerned about not eating his soup than having a transplant. It was actually funny when I think of that moment now. Then I called Jack. After telling him about the liver and the bile ducts he had me hold on while, once again, he checked with one of the transplant surgeons at Mayo Clinic. When he came back he told me it was a go. Soon we found ourselves back at the hospital with Michael getting prepped for surgery all over again He went through the same ritual as he had previously, with all the same tests. The coordinator was calling every couple of hours with updates. I phoned our shocked family and told them to be prepared. The time wore on just as it had the day before. Then the coordinator called. Very unflappably she apprised me of the situation, "Due to Super Storm Sandy, the plane along with the transplant team were unable to leave Cleveland to secure the liver." Once again there would be no transplant. That time the disappointment was overwhelming; much more so than the preceding day. Another dry run. Unbelievable! I was so shook up!

We left the hospital and went back to the hotel very down in the dumps and demoralized. Michael was in terrible shape due to having his meds discontinued two days in a row. Amy and I took care of him until he was better, and then she left for home. I was glad when the disappointing week was over. We were completely disheartened. The high spirits we had felt after Michael's acceptance were a distant memory. Adam joined us on Friday night for dinner and Darren on Saturday to help me watch over Michael and go grocery shopping. They mostly came to lift our morale. Our boys were a welcome diversion from a dreadful week. There is no question that the two dry runs had caused additional edginess to the already intense transplant process.

Chapter 23

THE WAIT

Mid-October to Late November 2012

Michael was feeling better by Sunday of the next week, so we had a car from the hotel take us to the local movie theatre. What a really lousy idea that was. He slept the whole time, not understanding or enjoying it for a moment. The bouts of encephalopathy had worsened considerably and had become more frequent. That particular day he really wasn't good, but he could do his little shuffle/walk, so I felt it might be nice to get him out of the hotel room. Thoughts of how much we used to like going to movies together on Sunday afternoons kept intruding on my concentration. After the movie was over we had the same driver pick us up and take us back to the hotel. The outing had exhausted Michael and caused me to be more despondent and lonely than usual.

I was looking out the window of the car, lost in thought, when my phone rang. A Cleveland area code showed on the screen. Again? Couldn't be! Not a chance! But, yes, it was another offer. I listened intently to the coordinator as she told me the liver was not compromised, however the donor was. Why was I not surprised? She said the person had passed away of an overdose, was an IV drug user, a prostitute and had tattoos that were of an unknown origin, meaning not professionally done. "You've got to be kidding me!" I said to myself, bordering on showing her my exasperation with the whole transplant process. Our coordinator then informed me that tests had been done and as far as the professionals knew, there was no disease, like Hepatitis C or AIDs, etc. She continued to say that they could not guarantee that any affliction related to the donor's lifestyle would not show up in my husband's body after transplant, but even so they all felt that was an acceptable risk.

The, "as far as they knew," statement gave me cause for alarm. Feeling very dubious, I took a moment to discuss it with Michael while she waited for an answer. He was cognizant enough to yell at me, "I don't want a druggie liver." Personally I was thinking, "We have had three offers in 10 days and Cleveland Clinic does approximately 150 liver transplants in a year." That seemed like a lot. I calculated, "If we don't take this one there surely will be another to take its place very soon." I, for one, didn't want Michael to trade one set of disastrous problems for another. The doctors at the Clinic had said he had less than a month and a half left to live; even so, I wasn't comfortable with that particular donor liver. Ultimately the mind-boggling decision was left to me. Calling Jack didn't seem necessary; my intuition told me I needed to say no and I did just that. Gambling with my husband's life absolutely terrified me. There was also worry as to how it would affect the chances of him getting a transplant. I referred my concerns to our coordinator who said that not taking the offer would not have an impact on Michael's standing when another liver became available. I wasn't so sure about that. How could I not be skeptical?

We had received three offers in less than the two weeks we had been on the transplant list. To us, it meant that another liver was eminent. At that time during our wait when the phone rang it would make me psycho as I would think, "This is it!" But as the days and weeks went sluggishly by I grew to be increasingly discouraged, wondering if the transplant was going to happen in time. I tried my Pollyanna act, but it did little to lift Michael's spirits. He became sicker and sicker and sadder and sadder, as I became more mopey by the day. We were told that more transplants happened on the weekends, which I thought was a strange thing for us to know. It did cause us to be especially hopeful when Friday would roll around. Then Monday would come and our anticipation would start once more. It was a cycle that kept repeating itself ad nauseam.

Since Amy wasn't working, she would visit during the week for a few days at a time; Adam and Darren continued to come on the weekends. In the very beginning of our stay in Cleveland I was able to leave Michael in the hotel room for short periods of time when the encephalopathy wasn't too bad. I had the hotel staff on alert and willing to check on him if need be even though I knew he wouldn't leave the room. I would call while I was gone to make sure he was feeling all right. The brief outings with my daughter were a great diversion for me. On one of those occasions I called and he didn't answer. I couldn't help but imagine the worst as I rushed back to the room only to find him sound asleep in bed. It was the last time I left him alone.

When Michael didn't have an appointment at the Clinic, he would stay in bed or on the couch much of the day and eventually all day without leaving. I would sit with him trying to keep busy while I watched him stare at the TV or sleep. I prepared breakfast and lunch on most days and usually picked up dinner from the hotel restaurant. We could have had room service, but to tell you the truth, if I didn't get out of the room at least once a day I would have gone bonkers. Instead of sulking around all evening, I would leave Michael for a half hour, go to the bar and have a drink with my fellow caregivers, while waiting for a carry out. That was my night out. That was it for entertainment. Yippee!

Time passed and our kids continued to take turns coming to visit. Michael's sister Wendy and his brother Ronnie with his wife Linda, came once in a while too. With their help I could take Michael out for short periods of time. That was always a very nice change in our otherwise unremarkable days.

The small hotel we called home had a lovely seating area in front of a large stone fireplace near the lobby. It was good for Michael to get out of the room for even short periods of time when he was able. One day I had brought him downstairs and left him by himself on a couch facing the fire, where he could stay warm. He was fast asleep in moments: head back, mouth open, tongue out. I found a computer in the lobby and made myself busy. When I went back to collect him he was still napping but he wasn't alone. I found him surrounded on all sides by an entire group of men from Kuwait who didn't speak English. He was part of their party but totally oblivious to it. Taking in the scene, I couldn't help but giggle.

Our routine changed one morning during that interim period. I awoke to find the look on Michael I had come to abhor. With a ridiculous expression on his face, eyes bulging way out and mouth hanging wide open, I immediately knew we were both in big trouble. It was the encephalopathy again, but so much more intense than it had been since we had arrived in Cleveland, reminding me of the occasions when I called EMS. He was staggering all over the place and it took a great deal of effort to control him. His degree of agitation was greater than it had been in the past. I lead him into the bathroom, getting him there in the nick of time. I asked him if he needed help and he nodded his head "yes," but when I tried to assist him he became angry, grabbing my arm and pushing me down on the floor. Of course, he didn't know what he was doing, but it was the first time he had shown any type of aggression towards me and I was concerned that it might be something new to look forward to. When he was finished with his business I pulled him with all my strength until I finally got him into the bedroom where I forced him onto the bed. He immediately crumpled into the fetal position, falling asleep.

Contacting his gastroenterologist/hepatologist was the only thing I could think to do. His suggestion was to call EMS and have him taken to the ER if I couldn't handle him myself. It was for me alone to decide and I just couldn't do that. My husband's health was so fragile then, I knew if I took him to the hospital it could be fatal. What if he caught a virus or some other disease while there? The fact that if he got any more feeble they might take him off the transplant list kept me from calling EMS. For two days I nursed him and fed him, not leaving his side. Gradually he started recovering. However, as usual he was not as good as he had been before the incident. He was absolutely horrendous, beyond anything I would have ever imagined. All the time I believed he couldn't get any worse until he did, over and over again.

During our last meeting with Cassie, she had given me the phone number of a couple, Jerry and Jill, who had been in our situation, waiting for a liver in Cleveland. He had been transplanted almost two years earlier. Jerry and Jill would be happy to talk to us if we chose. At first I didn't feel a need to share my experience with them. That changed on the days I was stuck in the room with Michael. When he was feeling better we called them. It was nice, especially for me, to talk to someone who knew some of what I was going through. Jerry and Jill became our friends. I don't think Michael got as much out of it at first as I did. I knew I could call Jill at any time for emotional support and later she found she could call me for the same support.

And so we waited! Our days kept turning into weeks and before I knew it a month was gone. It didn't take much for me to start questioning my decision in not taking the "druggie liver," as there didn't seem to be an end in sight to the waiting. I knew that sooner or later something was going to have to transpire; I prayed that it would be what we wanted. I was fearful that it wouldn't. Had I made a tragic mistake? I began thinking I had.

Chapter 24

THE CALL

November 27 and 28, 2012

November dragged on and on and on. I couldn't believe there had been three offers in a little more than two weeks after Michael's acceptance into the transplant program and then we heard nothing at all. My phone was way too silent. To give us some hope, we were told another statistic: on the holidays there were more transplants than at any other time during the year. Really? That kind of talk was very disturbing to me. Anyway, Thanksgiving came and went and we waited. We were at a point where we didn't even expect to get the call. It felt as though we would be in limbo forever.

On November 27, around 7 a.m. on Tuesday morning, I was awakened by a phone ringing. As I said before, I had become a light sleeper since Michael had been ill, so I woke up right away without a problem, but was still in a somewhat sleepy daze. My hubby, on the other hand, became conscious at a snail's pace. The phone rang and rang while I searched for it in the dark on my nightstand where I had been charging it the night before. I finally reached the phone assuming it was mine that was ringing, but suddenly realized it wasn't my ring tone. Then I thought it was the hotel phone. It took a moment until I recognized it was Michael's phone ringing, not mine or the hotel's, which was strange as he didn't receive many calls. Not for a minute did I think it was our transplant coordinator. She was in the habit of calling me, not Michael, as she knew he was plagued with encephalopathy. In the early morning darkness I watched as he leisurely picked up his cell phone and just stared at it, as it rang and rang. I scrambled over to him as I tried to get my hands on it while yelling, "Answer the f---ing phone!" He just continued to gaze at it, then casually handed it over to me. "Who could it be on the phone at such an early hour?" I thought, afraid to think it might be our coordinator. For the fourth time, with nervous tension and adrenaline surging through my body, I became charged as I heard her voice telling me they had an offer for Michael. I listened attentively as she recited the details. It was a very good offer and a better match than any of the others had been. The organ was coming from a young donor that had been in a car accident. At the time my feelings for the young person who had lost his life didn't register; those emotions would consume me at a later time. On that particular Tuesday morning I could only selfishly think of Michael and his life.

From what I was told on the phone I didn't need to call Jack to confirm we should accept the offer. I had become somewhat of an expert when it came to offers of livers for transplant, and this was the best one we had thus far. Besides, I knew Michael did not have long to live without the surgery; we were very desperate. I said, "Yes!" immediately without thinking or discussing it with him, feeling all the time that maybe my gamble of not taking the druggie liver had paid off. After receiving the usual instructions I woke Amy who was staying with us that day and we were off and running. Within an hour we were checked into the hospital and in a room. Of course, all the time I couldn't stop thinking that it could be another dry run. I prayed and prayed the transplant would take place and that we wouldn't be sent away again.

Our family was alerted of the pending event while Michael endured a plethora of tests. All meds were stopped and IVs were administered. By 9 a.m we were ready and waiting for the coordinator to call. She phoned around noon with no news and said she would be calling with an update every couple of hours. By 3 p.m. there was still nothing to tell us, except that the procurement team hadn't left Cleveland and she wasn't sure when that would happen. For someone who doesn't get perturbed a lot, I was doing my share. My darling man, on the other hand, patiently waited, only complaining he was hungry. At that point our boys, along with Wendy, Ronnie and Linda, had arrived.

Day turned into night and we were still on hold. The man in the next bed was very sick, so Michael sat at the end of the hallway with our family. He was so sweet during that time. It was the encephalopathy at work, but I welcomed it, as he seemed unaware of how dangerous the operation was going to be, and that he may die that night. It was amazing that he showed no concern and was actually having a good time with everyone. I can't say the same for myself as I walked up and down the hallways thinking the words "dry run."

After 6 p.m., calls from our coordinator became erratic. It was another déjà vu experience. I was expecting the calls to come every two hours and there was nothing. Thoughts of why my phone wasn't ringing besieged me. I could not take it if we were sent away again. At one point I didn't care about irritating her; surely she would understand how anxious we were. I called her; again she had no information and would call me back. Hour upon hour passed with no word.

Finally at 11 p.m. I saw the Cleveland telephone number light up my phone; this had to be it. And it was! She told me the team had just taken off in a plane to procure the liver. The transplant surgeon who would be doing Michael's operation had gone with them. The donor had been in a car accident and suffered some internal injuries causing trauma to the organ. The surgeon wanted to make sure himself that it was viable for transplant. That was something I hadn't thought of. Although I was glad he was checking it out, the call left me completely discouraged as it sounded like a potential problem. Great! Just great! She added that the process would take a while and I would hear from her later. I paced and paced the sleepy halls of the hospital, waiting and waiting. We all watched as helicopters took off and landed from the roof top of the building next door, saying to each other, "This could be the team!" Were they coming or going? We had no idea.

At 1 a.m. on, November 28, our coordinator made her last call to me. After having just spoken to the transplant surgeon she delivered the news I had been longing to hear: the liver was good. Although it had suffered some injury due to the accident, it was minor. The surgeon had been able to repair any damage; the rest would heal within Michael's body, as long as the transplant was a success. Incredible! Of all that I had learned from the transplant staff and in the class, the latest bit of information was over the top and hard for me to digest. I was also told that my soon-to-be-new hero was on his way back to Cleveland Clinic with Michael's gift of life. The transplant would happen within hours. No dry run this time! Michael would be taken to pre-op at around 2 a.m., with the surgery scheduled to start at 3 a.m.. My prayers had been answered just in time to save my husband's life.

Even though it was what I had been hoping and praying for, the fact that the transplant was imminent was terrifying. I can't say I was overjoyed or relieved, because I was so dazed and so afraid. I kept thinking that I needed to stay strong for Michael. I could not show him how I really felt. No way! He, however, did not exhibit the slightest bit of fear.

Chapter 25

SHOWTIME!
November 28, 2012

Suddenly, in the quiet of the night we heard the distinctive sound of the gurney rolling towards us. It was coming to take my husband for his life-changing surgery. Michael climbed on by himself without any qualms or apprehension of where it would be taking him. When it started to move, Amy walked along one side holding her dad's hand, and I walked along the other side of him, choking back the tears while trying with great effort to stop shivering. Our family followed behind us, caravan style, as we made our way down the dark hallways. A minute earlier we had been an animated bunch while we all tried to help each other keep our minds off what Michael was about to go through; following the gurney we had become a somber group. The buildup to that point had been incredibly stressful. I felt unprepared and not nearly as emotionally brave as I wanted to be.

After an endless trek through various corridors and elevators in the sleepy, still hospital, we found ourselves at the final destination. The door to the pre-op opened as we approached and we were met by a very compassionate OR nurse.

He gave us a few minutes alone with Michael. I stayed back letting the family have their time, lost in my own thoughts. I waited until they were finished, then hugged my vulnerable husband. We could each feel the other's love, the way we always had. Watching as they wheeled him away was extremely painful; there is no way I could possibly describe it. I completely fell apart, letting myself go, as I could no longer contain my feelings. I was in total shock and complete despair, thinking I may never see the love of my life again.

The whole family was experiencing similar raw emotions as we stood in the cold hospital basement, not knowing where to go or what to do next. The main surgical waiting room wasn't open at that time in the morning and the small room that had been assigned for family was occupied. There were only benches lined up against a wall in the freezing hallway. That's where we congregated, but only for a few minutes.

We were all startled by the same male nurse who appeared through the pre-op door again. There was a common thought among us: something was wrong, but we were wrong! They wouldn't be taking Michael into surgery for a while and the nurse didn't see any reason we shouldn't be with him since he was already prepped for the operation and there were no other patients in the pre-op that night. He escorted us into the large dark room, empty now, except for one lonely bed with a meager light above it. The whole thing was creepy, like a scene from the movie *Coma*. There lay Michael, all by himself looking very defenseless. In the dim light he appeared even more jaundiced and frail than he had earlier. As the family congregated around the bed, we could see his spirits soar.

I had asked the nurse if they would give him something to help him relax before surgery. He said a definite "No!" to that request. Actually, his ammonia-filled, mentally unbalanced brain seemed to be handling whatever stress he might be experiencing. Again, I wondered if he understood the gravity and seriousness of what was about to happen: that he could die that very night, or was he putting on a show for all of us? There was no way to know, but I didn't think it was an act and at that time I was glad he had the ghastly encephalopathy.

I don't recall what we talked about in that surreal setting, all I remember was meaningless babble. We hadn't been there very long when I saw a surgeon walking quickly toward the operating room wheeling a container behind him. I knew instantly it was Michael's gift of life. Soon the doctor came to introduce himself to his patient. Dr. Koji Hashimoto, an extremely charismatic and very confident surgeon, told all of us he had just flown in from somewhere he couldn't divulge and would be ready shortly to perform the transplant surgery. Michael, who had retained his wonderful sense of humor even though he was wacky as hell, asked the doctor if he might need a nap first, guessing he must have already been up for hours. Even then, at that seriously grave time, he sensed a tense situation and gave it some levity. It was one of those traits I had come to love about my wonderful man.

As Dr. Hashimoto walked away he turned to the nurse and said, "Let's go!" Once again, my heart did a flip-flop as I froze. Once again, the family one by one kissed Michael and said what they needed to say. And once again, I tried to hold back my emotions when it was my turn. The little boy that lives inside the man I love so much looked up at me tenderly and smiled. We kissed and hugged. Even though his mind was not all there, his heart was and I sensed all the love we had for one another. It was pure torture for me as we held each other and I felt the wheels on the gurney start rolling him away. I gave Michael one last squeeze. The scene was in slow motion as he was taken from me through the double doors to the OR. I tried like hell to not think that he may not survive, yet the thought was there all the same. He was almost out of sight from his family, when, surprisingly, Mickey got up on his elbows, turned his head around to look at us and said, with a huge smile, "It's showtime!" Then he disappeared around a corner. As long as I live I will never forget that moment.

I felt Darren's arms surround me, while the persistent aching pain and fear I had been living with erupted again from within me without restraint. The hysteria I was feeling was way too much to handle and I collapsed, shaking so hard I couldn't move. If the unthinkable happened to Michael, I thought my life would be over. Whether that was true or not, I can't say, but it was true for me at that moment. The torment I felt was more than I could bear.

As with the many things that happened that night, I don't recall how I ended up back in the hallway, but there I was with my family lined up on the uncomfortable bench in the cold hospital basement. The only memory I have is of sobbing and not being able to stop. I wanted to console my kids but I was unable. My mind would not stop repeating the thought, "I may have seen Michael for the last time; he could die!" Pollyanna was gone.

Chapter 26

WILL I EVER DANCE WITH MY HUSBAND AGAIN?

November 28, 2012

Sitting in the austere, drafty hospital basement was neither comfortable nor adequate. There were no restrooms close nor was there any place to get something to eat, not even a vending machine nearby. At that point I was beyond noticing where we were. As a caregiver I had been so occupied with Michael that thoughts of being concerned for my family or myself had become secondary. I knew they wanted to take care of me, so I gladly let them do just that.

It was 3 a.m. when Michael's OR nurse appeared in our waiting area to tell us the surgery had begun. I was in a state of shock. Just the sight of the nurse made me catatonic. Adam took charge, telling the nurse, "My mother cannot wait here for hours!" The sympathetic nurse understood as he looked at our family lined up against the wall. He had us follow him through a different maze of hospital hallways until we reached the main surgical waiting room, which had been closed earlier for the day. It had all we needed to make our long wait comfortable and we had the whole place to ourselves. The nurse left, promising he would call us in the waiting room with an update.

The first two hours were critical. The surgeon was going to look for signs of cancer when he started the operation. If he saw any, Michael would be closed up and not get the transplant. The liver would be given to another transplant recipient who would be prepped and on standby. Although, when I think about it now, there was no sign of another patient. My husband would surely die if they found any cancer. Adam was the only one in the room who had that information because he had been at our initial appointment with the first transplant surgeon. I had not shared it with the rest of the family, as it would only cause everyone more anxiety. Adam and I stared at the clock willing the first two hours to pass quickly. It was excruciating for me, as I was reminded of the pancreatic surgery.

My persona was somewhat composed by then, but even so I couldn't sit still; I paced and paced the large room as one hour soon became two. The nurse didn't call; instead he appeared back in person when the two hours were almost up. I held my breath while waiting for him to speak. The update he had from the OR was good; the surgery was proceeding and Michael was doing fine. Relief flooded through my entire body. I'm sure Adam felt it as well. We knew what that meant: no cancer.

The surgical waiting room was huge with various couches, chairs and tables throughout. All of us dispersed after the nurse left, each one finding a place to settle in for the long hours ahead. Adam found a small anteroom that doctors used for meeting family members after surgery. He was sound asleep within minutes. Amy and Darren were sleeping on couches at opposite ends of the enormous lobby, while Wendy sat at a table working on her computer. As for me, my pacing continued.

I tried to relax although it was a futile undertaking. When I wasn't worrying about the magnitude of the operation Michael was going through, my thoughts were of the donor and his family. It was not feasible to ignore their pain. As ecstatic as I would be if my husband survived the vital transplant, there would always be sadness for the life that was lost so that he may live. It hit me hard, as tears came when I remembered his loved ones and what they must be going through that very night at that very instant. Thinking about the transplant was acutely distressing, as someone had to pass on for our prayers to be answered. It was so very sad! I wondered how feelings about his donor would affect Michael. He didn't seem to grasp it before the transplant, but I was sure he would be as deeply affected as I was, and would always be, after he recovered.

At one point during my pacing in the dimly lit waiting room, a woman appeared from out of nowhere. Without prelude she asked, "What are you doing here?" and before I could answer she asked, "Is this all one family?" and before I could answer the second question she stated with the utmost of authority, "You are not allowed to be in here!" Just what I needed: a bitch. I was close to tears as I tried to explain that the surgical nurse had brought us there to wait and that my husband was undergoing a liver transplant. Still, she was in no humor to listen to my explanation or give me any sympathy. It was an ungodly hour in the morning and we were the only ones in the large room. All that didn't matter, as the overbearing woman threw all the lights on, waking any of us who were lucky enough to fall asleep. She found Adam in his cubbyhole and yelled at him, "You are not supposed to be in this area! This room you are in is reserved for doctors meeting with family members." What in the world was she talking about? At that time in the morning there was no one there but us. I let her rant and went back to my worrying.

Later she took up her post behind the desk, then summoned me. She was ready to take my name and give me a beeper, so I could get reports from the OR in a timely fashion. We hadn't heard anything since the nurse had given us the first report, and I was eager for any bit of news. Rudely she told me to wait for the beeper to go off, as it would give snippets of information from the operating room. She would give me nothing, nor was she inclined to call the OR for me. By now everyone was awake. Amy, upon hearing what happened, thought she could handle the situation given her social work training and went up to the desk for an update. The incivility continued and Amy returned with no news. Then it was Wendy's turn. If anyone could handle the bossy woman it would be Wendy. I'm not sure what she told the bully, but it worked. We were soon getting information regularly. The reports were all positive. Michael was handling the surgery well and everything was going as planned. Even so, I went back to my torturous contemplation and speculation.

Hour upon hour the emotional pain was persistent. I would make it through one hour and then would have a new one to deal with as the minutes ticked slowly by. The longer we waited, the harder it became to have a positive attitude. I couldn't help but envision what Michael's body was going through, yet it was impossible to actually comprehend. There was no reading or napping or TV for me, only clock watching and staring at a reader board which showed Michael still in the OR, as the anguish and tears continued. Thoughts of what our life had been like filled my mind: being together with our grandchildren and their families, living on our beautiful boat, all the wonderful traveling we had done and on and on. I thought about how Michael loved me. I could not live without that love; I could not live without him. How I longed to feel his arms around me again. It had been so long since I had that feeling. I imagined us on the dance floor laughing. I couldn't help but think, "Will I ever dance with my husband again?"

It is important to note, when there was some normalcy to my life, Adam and I contacted the Ombudsman office of Cleveland Clinic to report the woman who had behaved toward us without an ounce of compassion. I didn't want another family to have to endure what mine had during such a stressful time. The whole period we had been at the Clinic we all had been treated with utter kindness and consideration, so I knew that the hospital would want to know what had happened that day in their surgical waiting room. The person who took my call was so very grateful for the opportunity to address the incident. I have no doubt it will not happen again.

Chapter 27

LOUIE
November 28, 2012

In the quiet of the early morning hours my phone rang. Ordinarily I wouldn't have paid attention to it during the midst of a crisis, but I recognized the Chicago area code. Since that's where I am from, curiosity got the best of me, so I answered. It was the Northwestern Hospital Transplant Center calling. The appointment to review Michael's case had not been kept when Cleveland Clinic had put him on their list and their transplant team was calling to reschedule the examination. They wanted to assess him for their program. I gladly told the woman on the line that they were too late, as my husband was undergoing transplant surgery as we spoke. She was shocked and told me that it was the first time that anything like that had ever happened. It was a pretty weird moment to get that phone call.

The morning hours brought more and more people to our waiting room. I realized we had been at the hospital for over 24 hours. Was I tired? If I was, I didn't feel it. The surgeon hadn't told us exactly how long the surgery would take, although I knew it would be a lengthy ordeal. Still, after six hours we were all getting nervous. At nine hours, I was crazed with misgivings, though all reports from the OR continued to be reassuring.

At 3 p.m., 12 hours after the surgery began, it was finally over. We were given the wonderful news that Michael had survived. A while later Dr. Hashimoto found us in the waiting area. Beaming, he told us how well the transplant had gone. Michael's new liver was working perfectly. He had discovered the old liver to be shrunken, shriveled and not likely to support him for very much longer. Later he would inform us that Michael would not have lived for more than another two weeks. I hugged Koji as if he were my best friend, sobbing and thanking him at the same time. He was charged up after completing the successful surgery and appeared as if he had just slept 12 hours instead of operating for that length of time. In fact, Adam joked with him, "You look like you could do another one!" He joked back, "I'm ready!" We all encircled the outstanding surgeon, starring in admiration at the man who had saved my husband, their father and brother.

For the first time in a very long time I played with the possibility that Michael was going to be OK. It scared me to think that way. Needing to be ready for the worst had become a way of life. Can anyone ever prepare for an unhappy conclusion? Probably not. I certainly wasn't thinking straight after all we had been through. I wanted to be convinced we were past the second test of our lives, though I knew there was a long road ahead of us.

We were told Michael would be taken directly to an intensive care unit for liver transplant patients and there we would be able to see him in a couple of hours. The family all had people to call who cared about Michael and knew what he was going through; we each took some time to do just that. I could hardly speak I was so emotional. The most important call for me to make was to Michael Roth. Without his advocacy Michael would not have had his transplant. He cried genuine tears of joy, as I knew he would, when I told him about the miracle that happened at Cleveland Clinic that day.

Amy was especially sad as she thought of the donor. It hit us all at different times; that was hers. Our social worker appeared and was able to help her address the emotional up and downs she was feeling. It was hard to feel happy when someone you love was spared and another life was lost, in spite of the fact you didn't know him. Anyway, I was glad Cassie was there for my daughter, as I was a weary wreck myself and couldn't be of much comfort for her.

After some time we relocated to the ICU waiting room. Finally, 18 hours after I had said goodbye to the man I love, with thoughts of not ever being able to see him again, I was allowed in to visit. Usually I am not a take-charge person, but on that day I had no problem telling everyone that I would be going in alone. One at a time a family member could join me after I had my time with Michael.

Who would look good after one of the hardest surgeries a person could have? Nevertheless, I wasn't prepared for what Michael looked like. I knew he would be on a respirator and I knew about all the tubes that would be running in and out of his battered body and I knew about all the IVs. However, he was so swollen that he was hardly recognizable. I lost it and sobbed uncontrollably. My poor baby! I really couldn't take much more; he looked like he'd been beat up and tortured. The kind nurse who was taking care of him calmed me. She tried to assuage my fears, explaining that he had been given tons of fluids during surgery and that it would start to dissipate by the next day. After the initial shock I pulled myself together. Though Michael was unconscious I kissed him and talked to him, thinking he may know I was there.

Soon the family came in one by one, as I had requested. Amy didn't last a minute. Even though I explained the fluid retention, she took one look at her dad and went running. Our boys and Wendy could handle it better. Each one spent as much time with us as they wanted. Adam thought Michael looked like Don Corleone when he was hospitalized in *The Godfather*. I was sure Mickey would think that funny when he became conscious. We stayed in the ICU waiting room, going in to see him when it was allowed. At around 8 p.m., his nurse sent us back to the hotel.

We hadn't eaten much that day and needed to unwind, so we went to the bar. It was the very place where we had gotten the call that Michael had been accepted for the transplant program at Cleveland Clinic those many weeks earlier. After a short celebration, Wendy got a room and the kids and I had a slumber party in my room. I fell asleep thinking of Michael and his gift of life that we would soon come to know as Louie. Did I dare entertain the thought that Michael was going to come back to me?

Chapter 28

CRAZY MAN

Late November

The family was back at the hospital early the next morning. Again, I was shocked when I saw Michael, but in a positive way. As the nurse had assured me, the fluid retention, although still there, was not nearly as evident. What really surprised me was his coloring. For months his body and his eyes especially had been getting progressively more jaundiced. The day after his surgery his skin was pink and the whites of his eyes were actually white instead of the awful yellow they had been. In addition, I could see by the bag hanging on the bed that his urine was a normal color too, after being dark orange for as long as I could remember. It was like witnessing a miracle. Another surprise was that he was wide-awake and extremely upset with the tube in his throat. For some reason he thought I was the one who could get it taken out. I had expected him to be still out of it and drugged, yet he was just the opposite, wanting to talk or yell at me about the tube.

I was thrilled that he was angry. It was the first bit of emotion I had felt from him in months. He was trying to converse, as he waved his arms wildly in the air, but it all came out of him in grunts and squawks. Adam got him a clip-board and he immediately tried to write. The first thing was, "tube out". That we knew. Then he wrote, "wife cut me". What the in the hell did that mean? He wrote it over and over again. We had a hard time not laughing at him. Then I realized that a couple of days before I had cut his finger while giving him a manicure. Funny that he wrote that of all things. "Yogi", was the next request. Really? How did he expect to eat yogurt while still on a respirator?

Later that morning most of the family said their goodbyes and headed home with promises to be back soon. Amy stayed behind. Now that Michael was starting the recovery part of transplantation, she was there to help in any way she could and to keep me company. We stayed at the hospital all day, going into the ICU to be with him when permitted.

During rounds, the doctors told me Michael was doing well with no signs of rejection. That became my first worry during the early days after surgery. It had been talked about in the class we had taken. At the time it hadn't regis-tered as something I needed to be too concerned with, as all I had cared about then was getting him on the transplant list. All of a sudden it was of major rel-evance. I was told that it was normal in the days after surgery for the body to reject the new organ and that it could generally be handled with medication. That did not convince me that it wouldn't be a major consequence, especially since blood was taken regularly to check for it. It seemed the doctors were expecting his body to reject the new liver. The past several months my worries had been about one issue after another. I felt that if rejection were to occur after all we had been through, it would be more catastrophic than anything else that had happened thus far.

The next day the respirator was taken out, which made a huge difference since Michael could then verbalize everything he was thinking and, oh boy, there was a lot. And it was all twisted and mixed up. So much was going on in his head it was hard to sort it all out. That became my second worry. It seemed he still had encephalopathy. The doctors told me it would take some time for the ammonia to work its way out of his brain. The rest of the craziness, they promised me, was due to the surgery and all the meds he was taking. It was a combo problem that required my patience. I was getting more than my share of assurances that everything was normal when I felt it wasn't.

In the meantime, it was up to Amy and me to handle the wild visions Mickey was experiencing. First, he told us there was a Syrian general in the bed across from him. He kept making a motion with his hands, indicating the man had a machine gun. He was also on the lookout for the rest of the army. He was obsessive about the situation and told us, "Don't let them know I'm Jewish!" On one of our visits, we found him freaking out about flying golf balls, of all things. The following day Michael motioned around the small area at the numerous machines and IVs with their poles and bags hanging, asking me, "What kind of schlock place did you bring me to? It looks like I'm in a garage." He had no idea where he was. That same morning, he claimed, as if he was telling on them, "The nurses were having a party last night behind one of the curtains." He wanted them reported to the authorities immediately. On his third day he saw some Amish people visiting a family member and thought I'd taken him to the country. The patient in the next bed was making him nuts too. The lady kept crying out and he kept answering her as if they were having a conversation. To make matters even more confusing for him, his bed was across from the nurses station, so the intercom was something else for him to contend with. When it would buzz and someone would ask if they could visit a patient in the ICU, he thought they were talking to him and he would yell back, "Come in!" as loud as he could. When one of his doctors came to see him wearing his physician's coat, Michael thought it was a ghost or an image in a white flowing robe. Those were the visions I knew about; I'm sure there were others. He was very serious about all his hallucinations. Amy and I would have to turn our heads, so he wouldn't see us cracking up, as it was really funny. We couldn't help it; Michael was hilarious.

On the fourth day after surgery Michael was doing so well physically that he was moved to a room. It was a great change after being in the chaotic ICU. I was hoping that the relocation would help improve his mental status. At that time in his recovery he was really a crazy man!

Chapter 29

ONE STEP BACKWARD
Early December 2012

I had been impressed with the attentiveness shown to Michael in the intensive care unit. Not only was the staff extremely experienced in their various jobs, from the top doctors and nurses, to the technicians and therapists, to the aides and housekeepers, but also every one of them showed compassion and sensitivity toward Michael and me. It was amazing, with all they had on their minds and all their many duties, that they found time to show empathy for our situation whenever they could.

Given our wonderful experience in the ICU, it wasn't surprising that I was uneasy when Michael was moved to a private room. I knew it might help him mentally to be in less hectic surroundings, but would the staff there be as vigilant? Would I need to spend the nights with him? No worries; they were fantastic from the very beginning. The head nurse on the floor was there overseeing everything from the time we arrived. There was no annoyance shown at my slightest request, making me feel I could come to him for anything. It was comforting that all the nurses and aides were so accommodating, because physically Michael needed a lot of attention and mentally he needed even more. My hubby isn't a great patient with the slightest of colds, so you can imagine how he might react after major surgery. He required nonstop tender loving care from the nurses, the aides and from me. Amy was still there to share the burden for another day.

It took a while for the move to the new room to be completed. It was not a simple chore as Michael was connected to all kinds of equipment: a tube in his nose taking care of stomach gases, more than one IV bag, the catheter and its bag of urine, a heart monitor, various types of drainage tubes around the surgery sight connected to even more bags, a connection to an oxygen tank and a compression apparatus wrapped around his legs to stop blood clots. There could have been even more. Some of the things he'd been connected to had been taken away already, but there was still a lot to go.

Once settled in his new environment, it was time to get to work. Michael desperately needed to move around. He hadn't been out of bed since he was first admitted to the hospital, and he was in a wheel chair before that. His first task was to sit in a regular chair. His nurse and aide who came to move him had their hands full. It was painstakingly slow traversing the short distance. How great it was seeing him do a simple thing like sitting. Except for the goofiness he was exhibiting, Michael was really making progress and, so far, there wasn't the slightest sign of his body rejecting the new liver. Every day I became more hopeful that he would have a complete recovery.

We had a different transplant coordinator visit us when we moved to the new room; she would be our fourth. Who would have thought that there would be so many? I called them my "angels" because they were there whenever Michael or I needed assistance. Number four's job was to see us through the hospital stay, help get the meds organized and get us ready to be on our own. I had found out that all the angels were nurses, which was very reassuring, especially because the latest one would be teaching me about Michael's home care. She had brought with her an enormous tin box. I found out why it was so large when I looked inside. It was filled with prescription bottles of all shapes and sizes along with instructions on how and when the meds were to be given. Our new coordinator informed me that my job was to be with Michael all day, every day while he was in the hospital, as I would be the one to administer his medication and learn to take care of the surgery site. Really? I was counting on the nurses to do all that. At first I thought it was absurd. I could hardly look at Michael's wound let alone take care of it and, as for the pills, they were keeping him alive and great attention was needed in how and when they would be given. I was a virgin at the whole transplant thing and, after all, we were in one of the top hospitals in the country. Why wouldn't a professional be the one to perform the nursing duties?

In hindsight, it was good that I had to undertake the huge obligation, as I would also be required to do it when we got out of the hospital. The nurses were with me, giving me assistance and instructions every step of the way. I was advised that learning with the staff would inevitably make it easier on me when Michael and I were alone, so I rolled up my sleeves and started my education. Even though I had read about all the medications in the box, I was still relieved when the in-house pharmacist paid us a visit and explained each of them to me. I was taught how awful the lifesaving drugs could be. The side effects alone were very scary and the correct timing of their doses was essential. I would be responsible for giving Michael the right meds in a punctual manner. They were keeping him alive, so the job was daunting for me. The whole process of learning about the medications did not come easy, but in the end, with the help and unwavering guidance of the nursing staff, I became quite proficient with the assignment. It was days before I eventually knew all the drugs, their doses, what they were for and when to give them. I learned to take care of the large scar on Mickey's abdomen. The staff called it the Mercedes, because it was shaped like the car emblem. It was difficult for me to tend to. I was afraid of hurting him and doing it incorrectly, but I did it anyway.

The day after we got into a hospital room I sent Amy home to her family. She said goodbye in the morning. I would miss her most at night when I went back to the hotel; that was my lonely time. During the day I was very busy with my nursing duties and I was so overjoyed to have Michael back in my life that I loved staying with him as much as I could.

During his lunch that very day I noticed a subtle change in his mood. He was acting erratically. Was it the encephalopathy? No, it was different. He was usually more complacent during those episodes. He was acting disagreeable, extremely agitated and very jittery. Without asking for help he was trying to get out of bed, taking with him all his connections. He pushed me out of the way as I tried to calm him. Something was really wrong! Just then a respiratory therapist came in to check his oxygen, which gave me the opportunity to get his nurse. I got no further than the door when an alien-like scream came from Michael. I have never heard such a shrill screeching sound before, and the fact that it was coming from my husband terrified me. Racing back into the room I could see he was in the throes of a seizure. With panic clutching me I ran to the hall and yelled, "HELP!" as loud as I could. At the same time the much calmer technician hit the emergency call button located in the room.

They came from everywhere: all available doctors, nurses, aides and staff members. As the crash cart came flying into the room, I was unceremoniously pushed out of the way into the hall. Hysterically, I crumpled against the first person that touched my body. I didn't know at the time that it was a kindhearted nurse who was assigned to look after me. She led me to a waiting area, explaining on the way what was happening to my husband. I sat for a few minutes, gathering my strength back. She tried to stop me as I stood, but there was no way I wasn't going back into Michael's room. I had to see what was going on, I had to know he was alive. Trembling so badly I could barely stand, I ran back. The room was so jam-packed I only got a peek at Michael's pale face. He appeared to be breathing and the seizure was over.

Dr. Charley Winans, the transplant doctor in charge of Michael's case, took me aside. He told me that Michael was OK, but still in danger. As a precaution he was having him moved back to the intensive care unit immediately. He had been taking care of Michael and I knew him to be an extremely intelligent, compassionate surgeon with good judgement. Whatever he decided would be the best for his patient.

Our current angel arrived almost immediately after the seizure to mollify me. She said that once the doctors stabilized him, Michael would be taken to the ICU where he would be watched more closely and seen by a neurologist for his new malady. As soon as I regained my composure I called Amy, who was almost home. She immediately headed back to Cleveland, promising to call the rest of the family. There was no way I could talk on the phone just then. All I could do was sit tight and think. I was paralyzed with fear.

The understanding social worker on the floor was there for me, feeling my agony and stress. There was no question I had taken the setback badly. It did help to talk about what had happened, although truthfully, all I wanted to do was see for myself that Michael was all right.

At last, I was allowed into the ICU. He was, as the social worker had assured me, conscious and alert although tired from the experience of the seizure.

Charley suspected, but couldn't be sure, that it was a result of the heavy duty medications he was taking. Even so, the neurologist, who had been called in as a consult, wanted a 24-hour EEG to rule out anything else.

When I came back later, my hubby's whole head was covered with electrodes. It was obvious to me they were looking for another problem, this one in his brain. I prayed they didn't find anything. Michael seemed stable at that point and smiled at me when I came into his cubicle in the crowded ICU. I got a chuckle when I looked at my nutty guy with his greasy hair sticking out every which way and the electrodes protruding from all over his head. He looked so silly. Seeing that he was fine and having Amy back by my side, I instantly started to feel better.

The next day Michael was back to normal, or at least his form of demented normal. The EEG results were good, so no concerns there. Except . . . what if he had another seizure and I was alone with him? That made me exceedingly nervous. In any event, we added a neurologist to the list of doctors we would be seeing for a while.

I had put all my trust in what the professionals told me. They had all concurred that the seizure was but a blip in the long recovery process and not to be given a second thought. However, I couldn't help but contemplate what the horrific step backward would mean to my husband's recovery and wondered if the rest of my life would be filled with one alarming incident after another. The last one was so unforeseen. Never had seizure been mentioned, leaving me with a feeling that there could be other unexpected events in the future to contend with.

Chapter 30

THE BOYS ARE BACK
Early December 2012

Two days later Michael was deemed out of danger by those in charge and released from the ICU. He was taken to another new room and deposited in bed, where Amy and I were left alone with him. He should have been somewhat comfortable, but he wasn't. He told us there was something bothering him as he wiggled around in bed. It wasn't the site of the surgery that was causing the trouble. It was something else. We kept adjusting the covers and his legs for him, thinking it was his imagination, as he was still pretty dopey. He had been off pain meds because of the seizure, only taking Tylenol when needed, so it wasn't surprising he was having some discomfort. Because of the hundreds of stitches and staples, he couldn't move too much without his abdomen hurting, but even so, it was amazing to us that he didn't complain more about pain after what he had been through. The new annoyance he was grumbling about wasn't pain, so we didn't take it too seriously.

First on Michael's agenda when he got back to a regular hospital room was getting out of bed again. Another stint in intensive care had set him back considerably. His nurse and aide carefully moved him to a chair for his first bit of exercise. As he started to sit down he shrieked at the top of his lungs, "What the f--k am I sitting on?" Everyone froze for a split second then the brave nurse lifted up his gown to check out what was under him. At that point Amy went tearing out of the room.

Oh no! The boys were back! It was The Twins again and this time they were so gigantic they were one, the size of a large melon. The boys were so swollen that Big Jim was nowhere to be seen. The only evidence of Jim was the catheter poking out from the very large Twins. As usual, Michael was beside himself with worry over the new phenomenon. When it came to his boys having an issue, it was always an emergency. The nurse tried to reassure him that it was not unusual. He would not listen to her and insisted his transplant doctor be called to his room ASAP. His aide helped him get up, trying to support the boys as he wobbled back to the bed. What a sight it was. By the time Charley arrived, my man was extremely unhinged. He wasted no time whipping back his covers exposing The Twins, wanting him to be as upset as he was and magically cure his latest problem. "What is this about?" he yelled at his very calm doctor. Charley merely said, "It is very normal! All fluids that you were given during surgery have caused the swelling."

Poor Michael was not in good way. Shortly, his aide appeared with a solution. She had fashioned a small pillow out of a towel to cradle the boys while Michael was in bed. Unceremoniously she placed the cushion under them. Later a sling was delivered to alleviate the discomfort when he began walking. However, The Twins were so enormous that they didn't fit into it. It was not a good day for Mickey or his boys.

His humor wasn't much better the next day. They took the catheter out, so there was another challenge that lay ahead. He was not allowed out of bed and sitting up was hard for him; he would have to urinate while lying down. Again his aide came to the rescue, devising a special urinal. It was not an easy task for

Michael, even with the new invention. We waited all day for the urge to occur. Late in the afternoon he thought he could do it. However, given the size of The Twins, Big Jim was hiding. Michael's frustration was palpable. Everyone left the room while I helped him search for his missing pal. Finally, mission accomplished. What a relief, especially for my poor guy.

On to another assignment: pooping. Michael was too weak to make it to the bathroom, so a commode was brought to his bedside. The things that I thought were no big deal were anything but for Mickey. The commode sitting in the middle of his room irritated and annoyed him. Creating quite a fuss, he ordered it to vanish. He tried everything he could think of to get rid of the thing. Nothing he said mattered; it stayed where it was.

In any case, now that he had been on solid food for a couple of days, the event was imminent. I called his ever-patient aide when it was time. I wanted no part of what was about to happen and waited outside the room. The two of them were in there doing whatever one does in that situation when I heard a wail come from Michael. "Oh no, not another setback!" was my immediate thought. I couldn't help but sneak a look in to see what caused the commotion. Apparently, his boys were so gigantic that they got stuck under the lip of the commode during the middle of his pooping. It didn't take much for me to realize the commode was filling up too fast and The Twins were in danger of drowning. I took in the scene and then looked at the stunned expression on Michael's face. I will leave the rest of what happened that day to the imagination. It was outrageous to observe. The aide was nonplussed by the horrid circumstances and motioned me out of the room, as did Michael. I left happily as she ministered to my husband. She truly deserved a medal.

And so on it went from one problem to the next; some minor, some not so minor. After what we'd been through, nothing seemed major, at least, not to me.

Chapter 31

THE ANGELS
Early to Mid-December 2012

very morning when I arrived at the hospital I was happy to find my husband's condition to be improving. The physicians were monitoring his blood closely, always looking for an indication of rejection and checking to make sure the doses of the anti-rejection medications were at the right level. All the testing done in those early days after surgery came back perfect. Daily our transplant coordinator came in to check on Michael and remind me how amazingly well he was doing. She was my cheerleader.

Even though the transplant team was fending off potential problems, toward the end of Michael's first week in the hospital a new complication evolved. Both his hands developed a severe tremor. I was told it was minor, however, I was concerned the involuntary movement had to do with the seizure because it happened after that incident occurred. The doctors were of the opinion that it was more likely another symptom of the very strong anti-rejection drugs he was taking and that it would eventually subside as his body adjusted. Michael, not being a patient man, was horrified. He wanted the shaking gone immediately, as the annoyance of not being able to hold anything without dropping or spilling whatever it was had become intolerable for him. I felt that they needed to get a handle on the latest post-surgery dilemma soon, as it was causing Michael a fair amount of embarrassment and depression at a time when he needed neither. Hopefully, I thought that one of the adjustments to his meds would take care of the tremors.

At the same time I became more and more troubled that Michael's mental capacity wasn't improving at the same rate as his body. I knew I had been told that the encephalopathy could hang on for a few days, but when it became a week and he was still pretty screwy, I worried that maybe it would be permanent since his blood work showed no indication of a chemical imbalance. One sign that he wasn't getting better was that he couldn't seem to organize his words; they would become jumbled when he spoke. When a nurse was injecting a medication into his IV, he asked her if she was following the right protocol. We all knew what he meant, but the way it was said sounded strange. Our coordinator reminded me again it could be from the surgery itself and the drugs he had been given. Only time would tell.

In the daytime he wasn't too mentally unstable. It was when it got dark that all hell broke loose. The nurses had his bed on lockdown, arming it so he couldn't get up without a loud alarm sounding, just like when he was in Sarasota Memorial Hospital. That made no difference to the wild man; he would attempt to get out of bed every night. One morning when I walked into his room he couldn't wait to tattle on some nurses who had accosted him when he tried to get up. "Three blond nurses attacked me last night," he reported. "One of them had me in a headlock while the others tied me down!" Because of the compression device around his legs he was sure that he was being bound to the bed. Of course, that wasn't the case. On another occasion he called me at the hotel in the middle of the night, whispering in desperation, "They have taken me out of the hospital into the country. I'm in some farmhouse overlooking a road. You have got to come and get me out of here!" I was getting dressed to go to the hospital, as I pleaded with him to hit the call button on the bed. Just as I was heading out the door, his nurse phoned to tell me that he had settled down.

The good news was that he had picked up a phone to make the call and that was a first. The bad news was that he was a nutcase at night. "Not unusual," I was told. They call it "sundowners" in the hospital. I related it to the encephalopathy we both had suffered through the past several months. His body was healing, but his mind was not. It was but another reason I was so afraid that his cognizance had been permanently affected. All the appeasing did little to stop my uncertainty.

I knew we would be getting a new transplant coordinator when it was time to leave the hospital, but, as usual, I didn't want a different one. Each angel was special to us and we never wanted to change, however, that's the way the system worked. During the second week of recovery we were introduced to our fifth transplant coordinator; I was told she would be our final angel. Once home, our new coordinator would be available to us at all times. She would speak with us on a weekly basis regarding the endless blood tests Michael would have to undergo, their results and any other concerns that might pop up. Any need for medication adjustments would go through her, which seemed likely to happen during the first months after transplant. I was immediately drawn to her. She would be my safety net; my newest angel.

The patience and compassion all of the transplant coordinators showed both of us throughout the process was incredible. They were always available when needed. I am eternally grateful to all of them. They helped us through the many stages of liver transplantation, as well as one of the most difficult times emotionally in our life. Angel number five would be with us forever. I had no doubt she would be as attentive and caring as the several before her had been.

While in the hospital, Michael received the best possible care imaginable. I felt safe under their vigilance and was at ease. Thoughts of taking him back to the hotel and being on my own were frightening. I, for one, was in no hurry to leave, but as his health and stamina got better day-by-day I knew he would be released from the hospital soon. Having an angel always there for us made the thought of the transition easier.

Chapter 32

THE MIRACLE MAKER

December 12, 2012

By the end of the second week in the hospital it was evident that Michael was slowly coming back to me. Big Jim and The Twins had gone back to normal, he had regained enough strength to walk the halls without a walker (only holding my hand), the hated commode was gone, his appetite was great, and finally, after what seemed like an eternity, he started talking more sense than he had in many months. So much so that he wanted his cellphone. The fact that his mind was better made me the happiest of all. The tremor was still very bad and not showing signs of dissipating, but that was the only complication that he was dealing with.

Mickey was ready to get out of the hospital. On Dec. 12 he got his walking papers along with tons of instructions from the nurses. That afternoon we brought in lunch and goodies for the entire staff as a thank you for all that they had done for us.

We were elated when Koji came to check up on Michael before we left the hospital. He was undoubtedly very proud of the successful surgery he had performed. Every time I saw him after the operation I couldn't help but show my appreciation; I was in awe of his brilliant lifesaving skill. Now that my guy's mind was good, he wanted to give him a proper thank you for saving his life. His emotions were raw as he tried to put into words how he felt. As an afterthought Michael said to him, "You did a good job!" Koji, never at a loss for words, answered, "What are you talking about? I did a great job!" I loved hearing that.

We were waiting in the hospital room to be discharged when we had another unexpected visitor, Dr. Charlie Miller, Director of Liver Transplantation at Cleveland Clinic. I knew the minute I laid eyes on the man in the white coat that he was our miracle maker. In the end he was the doctor who made the decision to review Michael's case when no other physician or transplant center would so much as consider my husband. Northwestern had shown some interest but they had not assessed him. Charlie was the only one who had taken the time to know Michael as an individual by studying his file, he wanted to learn more about his medical condition and realized immediately he didn't have long to live. He was the only one not concerned with the protocols that other transplant centers abided by. He was the only one who really looked at Michael's life and gave him a chance to live. That day I knew he wanted to see, in person, the man whose life he had surely saved. Being so very grateful to him for giving my husband back to me, I couldn't help but hug the surgeon I had never met. Embracing him was so very easy for me and he embraced me back, confirming all the warmth I had expected him to have.

He settled himself in a chair and carried on a conversation with us as if he were not one of the busiest doctors at Cleveland Clinic. I know he could tell from talking to Michael that he had made the right determination by accepting him for a transplant. I'm sure he knew how deeply appreciative and grateful we would be for the rest of our lives. By listening to their banter it was evident that Michael and Charlie hit it off. As they conversed, you would have thought they had known each other for ages, especially when the conversation turned to talk of corned beef sandwiches and rib dinners. I had a feeling they'd be friends forever.

One of the greatest concerns of all transplant patients is the fear of rejection. I had been dealing with thoughts of it occurring since the surgery. Because of his debilitating mental state, Michael hadn't been dwelling on the subject. He was only just starting to focus on rejection, so he brought up the possibility of it happening with Charlie. With great conviction, Charlie stated, "Rejection will not be a problem for you!" Whew! I didn't care why he said it or how he knew it, I just loved hearing it. After all, he had performed and overseen hundreds of liver transplants. He didn't make all the anxiety go away, but it really did help.

As we continued to speak, Charlie noticed Michael's palsy-like tremor. Soon what had started as a social visit turned into a physical examination. He documented the tremor by taking a video of Michael's hands for the purpose of comparison. He would use it later to check Michael's progress. Seeing my husband struggling to pick up and hold things in his hands, Charlie felt it needed to be dealt with.

One of the best things about our new friend and doctor was that he believed in the quality of life. He could feel Michael's frustration concerning the shaking, which showed no signs of subsiding. Charlie exuded confidence when he ordered one of the anti-rejection meds stopped, feeling it was too strong for a man of almost 70. He made an appointment for Michael to see him at his office the next day, at which time he would have the stronger drug replaced with a milder one. It seemed Charlie was taking over his case. During Michael's stay in the hospital he had been seen by several of the transplant surgeons. It would be nice to only have one to go to in case of a problem. We couldn't have felt safer. Charlie left us with the assurance that the tremor would soon be history. I totally trusted and had faith in him!

As we left what had been Michael's home for two weeks we asked the aide pushing the wheel chair to take us on a loop of the hospital floor. We wanted to thank the whole staff for the fabulous care we had received. With qualms and nervousness, we said our goodbyes.

Soon we were settled comfortably at the hotel, feeling somewhat safe being so close to the Clinic. This would continue to be our residence for at least another month or more. We were especially happy that the miracle maker who had helped to give Michael back his life would now be his doctor and our new friend.

Chapter 33

ROCK STAR

Mid-December 2012 to Late March 2013

From the time we had arrived at Cleveland Clinic, our family took turns spending time with us and assisting me with Michael. That continued after we got out of the hospital. Their constant watchfulness helped my guy recover faster. Our grandchildren sent us pictures to decorate our room while staying connected to us by phone. During one of those conversations Michael's new liver was dubbed Louie and it stuck. It seemed to help the kids accept and be able to talk about the serious episode that had happened in their papa's life.

Once back at the hotel it was time to slowly start enjoying life again. Our first outing was no further than the hotel restaurant where I had friends that had only known Michael when he was sick. I wanted them all to see the change in him. Early on I had nick-named the cocktail lounge the Caregivers' Bar, as it had been my salvation with the many other caregivers that hung out there and especially with it's empathetic bartender, Jeff. That is where we went for our first dinner. Michael who was used to being the center of attention, especially with his new liver, expected a rousing welcome. He was more than shocked when my friends gathered around me instead of him. They had been there through my sadness to elation and were so very happy with our outcome, as it gave them all hope. Soon they gave notice to Mickey and showed him all the adoration he had been anticipating.

With Charlie's help and the support of our latest angel, Michael continued to thrive. Visits from a home care physical therapist and a medical nurse aided in his recovery and as promised, the annoying tremor was soon a thing of the past. All the incapacitating symptoms Michael had suffered from his liver disease were a bad memory. In fact, he no longer had alpha-1 antitripsin deficiency. It had left him when his liver was removed. Most important of all, with the terrible encephalopathy gone, we could communicate. It was such a simple thing and what I had missed most the last few months.

I thought we were home free when at one of his weekly appointments Michael complained of leg pain. Now what? He was sent for an ultrasound. They were looking for a blood clot and they found one. It was small and needed to be treated and watched. None of his doctors were terribly concerned about it and we didn't let it faze us, as we had learned to live with more disabling matters than a tiny clot. We just added a vascular doctor to the list of the many physicians we had accumulated. No biggie!

New Year's Eve was Michael's 70th birthday. Sally and Michael came to celebrate with us. It was a special birthday, mostly because he had been so close to death a month before, so I needed to get him something meaningful. I chose the smallest of charms for him to wear on the chain around his neck. On one side it said "Showtime", on the other, his new birthday: "November 28, 2012". I could tell by his tears how much my gift meant to him.

January dragged on with appointment after appointment and blood test after blood test. By the end of the month, Charlie was very satisfied with the progress Michael had made. It was time we left the safety net of Cleveland Clinic.

Michael and I were ecstatic with the thought of going home, even though there were great feelings of doubt and uncertainty. I, especially was secure being on the grounds of the Clinic. Now I would be on my own if anything happened to Michael.

Although he wore a mask when he was in crowds, we were paranoid about disease. Michael now had a compromised immune system due to the medications he was on. We also needed to continue taking precautions in regards to the blood clot and I was deathly afraid of another seizure. Of course, what if he had rejection? It was still one of our biggest worries, even though Charlie had been confident that it was something we need not be concerned about. We were assured that the transplant team, with their surgeons, nurses and coordinators, was a phone call away and would always be there for us. We said our tearful goodbyes and a sincere thank you to everyone and anyone we could think of at Cleveland Clinic and the hotel. I was taking my man home.

Once we were back in Longboat Key, the reception Michael received was amazing and heartwarming, so much so you would have thought he was a rock star. Our friends at the marina put up a huge sign welcoming Louie. Everywhere we went, people were so happy to see Michael and everyone wanted a piece of him. It was hard to say no to all the invitations we had, but the truth was that we didn't want to do anything except be together.

We reconnected with our local doctors and Michael continued weekly blood tests at Sarasota Memorial Hospital, where every Monday it would be collected. Some of it was tested there and the rest was mailed to Cleveland Clinic to be analyzed. At first the wait for the results was hard for us, but week after week the findings were all good, so we guardedly started to relax. Sometimes a number would be off. Our coordinator would call and we would have to redo the blood test. One number was especially troubling to the transplant team causing Michael to need an MRI to determine that his bile ducts were not blocked. Until we got the news that there wasn't a problem, we were very tense. Aside from that one time, Michael's health has been very good since our homecoming. The blood clot eventually became a nonissue as Michael continued to do well.

In March we were back at Cleveland Clinic for a four-month checkup. After three days of scans and testing, Michael saw Charlie, our miracle maker, for his follow up examination. He was happy to report to us that his patient was doing remarkably well.

Just when we were about to leave the transplant floor we ran into another one of my favorite docs, Cristiano Quintini. He had been the first one we met when being considered for the transplant list, the one who had promised Michael, "I'm going to get you a new liver and you are going to live forever." Cristiano was glad to see how well he was doing. Michael reminded him of what he said that day and added, "Now that I'm going to live forever I have to get a job." We all laughed at that.

Before we left the Clinic we made a special trip to the oncology department. We felt a sense of obligation to see the oncologist who had researched Michael's cancer case so thoroughly. He had given a positive report to the transplant committee and was a key figure in Michael's acceptance for transplant. In seeing the life he saved we hoped he would know how important he had been. The doctor humbly accepted our words of thankfulness.

Because he was such a success story, everyone wanted to see Mickey. Once again he walked around like a rock star. He should have worn a tuxedo, as it seemed everywhere we went he was walking on a red carpet. Cleveland Clinic had taken a chance on Michael and so far he was one of their superstars. The entire staff wanted to see their walking, talking miracle.

Chapter 34

THE DANCE
March to November 2013

houghts of all that we had been through had changed from an abhorrent fate to a painful memory. Did we really go through all that I had just written about? The reality of our ordeal was becoming obscure to us both and yet we knew it had happened. The experience had left a different impression on me than it did on Michael, whose recollection was really far from crystal clear. As I surveyed the past I recalled it all, but as time went on, it began to take on a sepia tone. My memories were indistinct, becoming unfocused and shadowy, a kind of blur in my mind. I knew that period in our life would never be forgotten, but it seemed to be finding a comfortable place where it could be coped with.

Michael continued to flourish as he got farther and farther away from his transplant surgery. The change in him was amazing to watch. Slowly, we tried to live without fear and to have a normal life. Normal life? Could I really just go back to having a normal life? Thoughts of the cancer coming back, the encephalopathy, the terrible seizure occurring again and the chance of rejection were and are still very genuine fears for me. Because of all that, it has been hard to give up my role as caregiver. If you can believe it, I really want to continue caring for my husband. First, I feel he has been somewhat blasé when it comes to taking his medication in a timely manner, making doctor appointments, and other pertinent decisions regarding his health. Second, there is no question in my mind that I do a much better job of handling it than he does. If there have been any problems in readjustment at all after his transplant, it has been that I have had a very hard time backing off from overseeing his health care, and Michael doesn't need or want me to do it anymore. It is something we both struggle with. In time he has learned to be more tolerant of my fussing, as he has begun to understand what I went through and I try to be more trusting that he will take care of himself in a responsible way. We are compromising, but it is a challenge that we both need to deal with daily. We love each other and appreciate what the other has been through, so there is no doubt in my mind that we will overcome this obstacle.

Michael recovered from his liver transplant and I had survived it without developing PTSD. It was time to write the hardest letter of my life. What could I possibly say to those who had lost a loved one, while my husband survived because of that very tragedy? I unabashedly wept as I wrote to our donor family. After I put my heartfelt feelings on paper I sent it to Cassie, our social worker, who reviewed it and sent it on to Lifebanc. From there it would go to a grieving mother, father, wife, son or daughter; I had no idea who. All I did know was that I felt profoundly sad for what they would endure for the rest of their lives. If they chose to accept my letter or whether they answered it would be up to them.

Michael continued to see Isaac and Aida from time to time. Their doctoring was very significant during the end of his liver disease and we will always be thankful for the many hours they spent trying to find a transplant center that would review Michael's case. Their great care of him continued when we got home and it has been a relief for me to have them close by. They both appreciate the picture of health Mickey has become.

Joel and Jeanne didn't have to wait to see Michael, as they run in to him quite regularly in the fitness center we all go to. Joel's skillful treatment of Michael in the ER at Sarasota Memorial Hospital and Jeanne's attentiveness to our needs while he was hospitalized helped us make it through some very dark days. They too are delighted to see how well he is doing.

Then there was Big Dog. If it weren't for his candid comments that day in the hospital I might not have moved in an expedient way to save my husband's life. He deserved a peek at the rock star too. One afternoon we stopped by for a visit with him. He was surprised and thrilled when he met the real Michael; not the encephalopathic one he had cared for in the hospital.

Michael no longer goes to Mayo Clinic and consequently no longer sees our dear friend Jack regularly for his health care. He had been the most instrumental doctor in the days of the pancreatic cancer and liver disease, but more than that he had become so very special to both of us. I continued to stay in contact with him through the whole time we were at Cleveland Clinic, before and after the surgery. Upon Michael's recovery he, too, reached out to Jack. We were especially glad when during the summer Jack came to Florida for a visit. I couldn't wait for him to see the transformation in Michael. His emotions were clearly seen upon laying eyes on his friend and patient for the first time in over a year. It was important for us that Jack could know that his contribution to Michael's wellness had ended so very favorably.

Soon it was the September after the transplant. We both knew it was time to fulfill an important obligation. It had been one year since Rabbi Brenner

Glickman had appeared in Michael's room at the hospital to pray with us during Rosh Hashanah. My husband was so very sick and he gave us the hope we desperately needed. The rabbi left us with prayer books that we had promised to return to his synagogue when Michael was well. At the time, any thought of him recovering from his terrible affliction was hard to imagine, but there we were 10 months after Michael's operation and he was back to living his life, just as the rabbi had predicted so many months before. The day before Rosh Hashanah, 2013, we packed up the books and headed to the synagogue. Nothing felt better than watching my healthy happy husband hand the prayer books over to the equally happy rabbi.

After so much had been given to us, we both felt the need to do something for others. It was perfect timing when Cassie called us from Cleveland Clinic asking us if we would be mentors for other individuals living through the same kind of struggle that the two of us had just survived. We eagerly anticipated the prospect of helping in any way we could, Michael as a transplant recipient and I as a caregiver. To this day there are several patients and caregivers that we speak to on a regular basis. We will always continue to reach out to those who may need our advice and support.

We feel immeasurable gratitude to Mayo Clinic for saving my husband from his deadly cancer, to Sarasota Memorial Hospital for taking care of him in the interim, and to Cleveland Clinic for saving him from his damaged liver. There have been so many caregivers along the way that I hope they will read this story and know what a significant part they have all played in our lives. Now it is our turn to contribute in a meaningful way. My first gift will be my accounting of our experience, as I have great hopes it can be used to help patients and caregivers alike.

What can I say about our children that I already haven't said? They have been and will always be there for us. It's kind of funny that now Michael is well, he doesn't require the constant attention they once gave him. He misses it and is not shy when he tries various maneuvers to get into the spotlight again. The kids have his number, that's for sure; it's become a game between them. I can't imagine how much harder it would have been without them by our sides. We hope they will always feel the deep love we both have for all of them. Without their dedication Michael would not be alive today. I trust that every one of them knows how important they have been and will continue to be in our lives.

Then it was Thanksgiving: Nov. 28, 2013, one year to the day after Michael's transplant surgery. How fitting that his new birthday fell on Thanksgiving that year. There was no question that we would spend that important day with our kids. Our grandchildren were all too happy to have Louie's birthday to celebrate with cake and ice cream. It has always been Michael's custom to have everyone say out loud what they are grateful for at our holiday dinners. When it was his turn to recite his thankfulness he really tried to get the words to form, but his emotions took over. It was the best Thanksgiving we ever had.

On a Saturday night, sometime after Michael's lifesaving surgery, we went to our favorite marina restaurant for dinner. Little did I know how special that night would become. When the music started to play, Mickey asked, "Would you like to dance with me?" One year earlier I thought that would not ever be possible, but there he was, alive and well and in living color, asking me to dance. Tears welled up in my eyes as he took me in his arms. My heart melted as though I were a teenager on my first real date. I was joyous beyond words. Thoughts of the night of his surgery entered my mind. At the time I had wondered if Michael would ever be able to dance with me again. It wasn't that long ago that he couldn't even stand, let alone waltz me around a dance floor.

How could I be happier than at that moment? The song was "Have I Told You Lately That I Love You?" by Rod Stewart. The words were so meaningful:

Have I told you lately that I love you?

Have I told you there's no one else above you?

You fill my heart with gladness, take away all my sadness, and ease my troubles, that's what you do.

I had the love of my life back. My first dance with my husband in a very long time meant the world to me as I remembered coming so close to never having it. We were ready to start living again.

The plan was that this is where my book would end. I felt that my dance with Michael was a perfect finish to our story. And then …

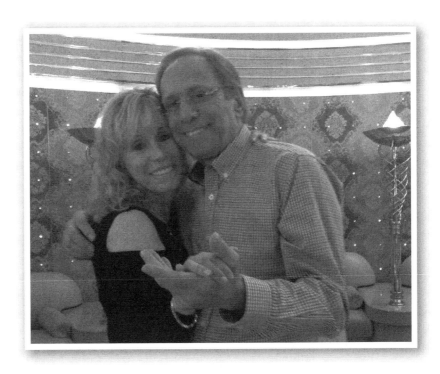

Possible Miracle

EPILOGUE
November 2013 to January 2014

And then . . . upon waking one morning I found Michael working frantically on his computer. Before I could ask him what he was doing he was off and running, out the door and over to the marina office. "I have to print something," he yelled as he headed out the door. I remember thinking, "What in the world is he up to?" When he came back he could hardly contain his excitement as he announced to me, "I just booked us on a world cruise for this January!" and flung the paperwork at me. His feelings were contagious as I flirted with the possibility of going on our trip of a lifetime. I had not so much as contemplated a grand voyage such as that, but there he was standing in front of me with his great smile. It was extremely infectious. He wanted me to be as jubilant as he was, so I simply gave in and was. Of course, we both understood that Michael's health would be the determining factor. There was no other option except to wait until his one-year check up, one month prior to the departure of our cruise. In the meantime, it wouldn't hurt to go ahead with the fun of preparing.

We were literally ready to leave on our journey when we went to Cleveland Clinic at the beginning of December. What was Charlie going to say? Would Michael be able to be away for that long? Even though he was doing great, I personally felt it may be too soon for him to go on an extended trip that took us to many exotic places. As much as we both wanted to travel, we knew that the decision would be in our miracle maker's hands; we would acquiesce to whatever he said, as we would never do anything without his blessing.

There was no point in putting the big question to him until after all the results from all the tests were compiled. At the conclusion of the examination we were waiting with anticipation when Charlie walked into the room. Without hesitation he announced that all was very good. Then, without preamble, Michael asked him if we could take a four-month journey around the world. I held my breath as I waited for our miracle maker's answer. Charlie looked directly into my husband's eyes and answered without equivocation, "Go on your trip around the world. We didn't save your life so you wouldn't live it!" He truly believed in the importance of the quality of our existence and knew the significance of this trip for us. His words astounded me for I knew at that extraordinary moment our nightmare was over and our precious life was truly back, along with a glorious future to look forward to.

The excitement we were feeling was of epic proportion as we approached the ship that would take us on our dream of a lifetime. How silly we must have looked, walking hand in hand crying like babies in the cruise terminal; we were so very giddy with emotion, as tears rolled down our smiling faces. Michael and I understood that our life had been reborn and without question we would eternally embrace and cherish our *possible miracle.* We are at a new place in our history with no doubt that there is nothing more life can throw at us that we can't conquer together. With an abundance of hope, prayers and courage we have made it through what has been the most difficult of times.

I realize as I write the finish to our story, there is no end, only many more beginnings…

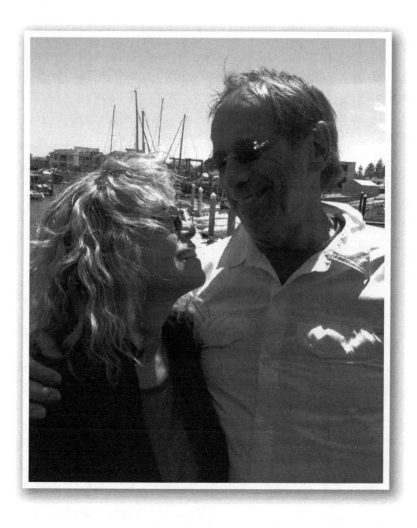

MICHAEL

Hi, this is Michael,

Quite a story and it's all true, no writer's privilege. It's very difficult reading something like this about myself without getting really emotional and almost not believing that the events actually could have happened, but they did!

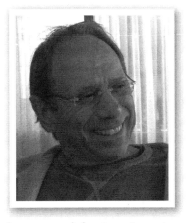

For many years I had a dormant condition now known as alpha-1 antitrypsin deficiency. I attributed little maladies that arose from time to time to it but never really took it seriously. Little did I know that it was going to have such a disastrous effect on me. While tracking the alpha-1, the pancreatic cancer was discovered. That was plenty serious. I can only be thankful it was found so early. Had I known about the BRCA2 gene mutation and about the enormous part my genetics were playing, I would have had a better understanding of what could happen. Then my liver went completely south and it was just about all over. If it weren't for things happening the way they did and for the help I received, I wouldn't be here today.

For two years or so prior to the liver surgery, everything is fuzzy. I remember only tiny snippets of things that happened and nothing of others. Of course, there were periods and even weeks when things went pretty well, but not many in succession. The bottom line is that I had no idea I was dying. I also believe that Susan becoming very proactive is what moved everything forward at warp speed. Had it not been for her along with Amy, Adam, Darren, Michael, Jack, Charlie and a few other very special people, I would not be reading our story or writing these words.

Clarity began around two or three weeks after surgery; ever so slowly my strength returned and my mind began to again function. It's been about two and a half years since I received my gift. I've discovered what's important in living and that priorities can change. Because of that, I do what I call "appreciations." I'm not talking about grandchildren, sunsets, travel, or smiles; they are obviously terribly, terribly valuable to me. I'm talking about appreciating people who selflessly help others and one such appreciation is for the role of a caregiver. I believe there is no job more needed by those who cannot do for themselves. Physically and emotionally, it would have been just plain impossible for me to have carried on for myself without Susan.

Regarding the transplant itself, I am not an expert and can only express my personal observations. In my case and, as in other survivors' cases I have run across, we have had similar experiences and feelings:

ENJOYING LIFE to the fullest,

ANXIETY about the process (I was really out of it as already discussed),

MIXED FEELINGS because I am living a healthy life with someone else's liver,

GRATEFUL to all the people and hospitals involved,

SLOWLY HEALING my anxiety-filled body and mind,

HELPING OTHERS in whatever way I can.

It's like having won the lottery of life. Time, family and friends, along with a good attitude are all so essential, as is asking for assistance. Following a plan, making it flexible enough for change and rigid enough to withstand that change is what helped me through the most challenging part of my healing.

I am so thankful for so many things and to so many people who have given so much to me. Especially I thank the staffs at various hospitals who brought me through my most perilous days, as well as our family and friends who helped and encouraged me back to health.

I found myself at Mayo Clinic and then Cleveland Clinic because they are world leaders in the treatment of many medical conditions as well as in research and education. Both are nonprofit and very large multi-specialty medical centers that are committed to the patients they serve. Mayo Clinic saved my life due to its diagnostic capabilities, but ultimately if it weren't for Cleveland Clinic's progressive practice of medicine I would not be alive today. To me these institutions retain a special culture of teamwork that make them extremely unique in the medical world. Their accolades are well earned.

At the top of my gratitude list is my donor and his family. It was one year after my transplant that I received an answer to the letter we wrote the donor family. I remember being afraid to open it at first as I knew it would unleash so many deep emotions. The letter was from a young father who had lost his 18-year-old son and it literally tore me apart. At the time I wasn't sure how I felt about having a connection with my donor family but as the letters continued I found comfort in communicating with the 40-some-year-old young man. In one of them he asked if I would be willing to email with him and soon we were conversing via email. In May of 2015 he asked if there was a way we could meet and he left his phone number. Without hesitation I called him and we set up a time and a date.

Susan and I were crazy with anticipation as the day approached late in May. The minute we saw each other there were hugs and tears as raw emotions came pouring out of us. As we talked he poignantly told Susan and I that the night of the car accident he stood at his son's bedside knowing that his prayers were not going to be answered and made the gut-wrenching decision to answer someone else's. He also candidly acknowledged that he had been initially upset at the age of some of the recipients but after meeting us his thoughts had changed. He could easily see how we lived our life and that it had been one he was glad he helped to save. As we said goodbye to him that day I took his hand and placed it on my belly so he could touch the part of himself that lived within me. We stood there crying and hugging one another. The feelings that I felt were such that I knew without a doubt we would be connected forever. Since that time we have had dinner together and plan to meet as often as we can. There is no question of the significant bond that has been formed. As Susan has so eloquently written, this wonderful and selfless act is the most genuine of gifts. I can only hope to do it justice by being there for this grieving father and by helping others.

We are more than happy to aid anyone who is contemplating a transplant, who is in the process of a transplant, who may want to be a donor, or who may need support in surviving an illness. Please contact us at **www.facebook. com/PossibleMiracle**.

Thank you for reading our story,
Michael Fayne

Possible Miracle

AFTERWORD

ichael's story is rather amazing from the medical point of view. He has survived four potentially fatal conditions: severe infant hepatitis, pancreatic cancer, primary liver cancer, and liver failure due to an inherited form of cirrhosis. I am sure that the pediatric surgeon who operated on a jaundiced, 3-month-old Michael was expecting to find an obstructed bile duct, but the operation report retrieved from the archives tells us that the ducts were wide open. Instead, a biopsy of the liver showed extensive liver cell damage and inflammation, a form of severe hepatitis that was caused, it turned out, by an inherited condition that was unknown at the time and only discovered more than twenty years later. Somehow, infant Michael survived long enough for his liver to regenerate, and he recovered. He stayed healthy through his adult life but eventually developed abnormal liver blood tests and—58 years after his first sign of liver disease—was found to have developed liver cirrhosis due to the same condition: an inherited variation in a single protein, alpha-1 antitrypsin.

I became acquainted with Michael and Susan when he landed in my liver disease practice at Mayo Clinic. I saw him at regular intervals over the next several years to monitor his liver condition. Many patients with cirrhosis maintain good liver function and normal activity levels, but they are still prone to developing changes in the liver cells that may turn into primary liver cancer, so the practice is to get a new scan of the liver a couple of times a year. Michael did some of the monitoring at home, but he checked in with us once a year in Minnesota. I could not help responding to his charismatic and outgoing personality, and we gradually became friends outside the office. My wife Julie and I would look forward to Mike and Susan's visits, and the four of us would usually go out to dinner.

It was during one of Michael's monitoring visits that the liver surveillance scanning incidentally showed a cyst in the pancreas. Although this initially looked innocent, further investigation showed that it was a primary pancreatic cancer. In most cases, cancer of the pancreas carries a dismal prognosis. However, we were fortunate to have found Michael's cancer in an early phase, and his subsequent surgery, combined with a protracted and difficult course of radiation and chemotherapy, gave us optimism that he had a good chance to survive.

We were less than three years into follow-up for Mike's pancreatic cancer when surveillance finally turned up a small primary liver cancer. We were able to use a microwave probe to kill the cancer cells directly, but the handwriting was now on the wall: if the cirrhotic liver had already formed a clone of malignant cells, it could easily do so again in the near future. In addition, Mike was showing signs of progressive liver failure, including disabling fatigue, massive fluid retention, and problems with thinking and disorientation secondary to the increasing toxins in the blood. The only answer was a liver transplant. The hooker in Mike's case was that most transplant centers would not consider putting in a new liver unless it had been at least five years since treatment for cancer. Unfortunately, this was also the policy at Mayo Clinic. Despite aggressive lobbying on Mike's behalf, I was unable to convince the transplant committee that three and a half years without evidence of recurrent pancreatic cancer was long enough. This was one of the greatest frustrations of my career. Even though I was not personally responsible for the decision, I felt like I had failed my friend Mike.

What happened after that is an inspiring story, and a testament to Susan's unfailing courage, steadfast love, and dogged persistence in the face of unacceptable odds. It is also an illustration of how a patient, no matter how bleak things look, may win through by maintaining an unconquerable spirit and a sense of humor. Michael now looks, feels, and acts like he is twenty years younger. In an earlier phase of his life, he developed and eventually sold a successful company; now he says he's thinking about starting another one. Godspeed, my friend.

Jack Gross, MD
Emeritus Associate Professor of Medicine
Mayo Clinic College of Medicine
Division of Gastroenterology & Hepatology
Rochester, Minnesota

Possible Miracle

HOSPITAL RECORDS

The following pages are from the 1943 archives of Boston Children's Hospital. The pediatric surgeon who operated at that time did not have a diagnosis thus Michael's surgery was considered exploratory and experimental.

5·365-121)   271023

NAME   Michael Fayne   No. A

DATE   March 27, 1943   AGE

PRE-OPERATIVE DIAGNOSIS   Cirrhosis of liver

POST-OPERATIVE DIAGNOSIS

OPERATING SURGEON   Dr. Gross

ASSISTANTS   Dr. Duncan. Dr. Rydell

TYPE OF OPERATION   Exploration of bile ducts. Biopsy of liver

DESCRIPTION OF OPERATION _____ (TO BE WRITTEN OR DICTATED BY OPERATING SURGEON)

OPERATION RECORD

General anesthesia. Right rectus incision retracting the muscle
laterally. On entering the abdomen the liver was found to be
greatly enlarged and to have a greenish color. There was, however,
almost no dimpling of the surface to suggest scarring in the
underlying liver tissue. The findings were more compatible with
an acute hepatitis than they were with a cirrhosis of the liver.
The gall bladder was normal in size and appearance and contained a
few c.c. of bile-stained fluid. The cystic, hepatic, and common
ducts all appeared to be intact and apparently patent as far as I
could tell. A catheter was sewed into the gall bladder and
saline was injected. This showed definite patency of the cystic
and common ductus, because fluid flowed down into the duodenum.
The hepatic duct likewise seemed to dilate during this procedure.
At the end of operation I was inclined to believe that the patient
had no actual obstruction of the ducts (unless there was some plug
which I dislodged). Changes seemed to be more consistent with an
acute hepatitis of some sort. The opening of the gall bladder was
closed with a circular silk suture, the abdominal wall was closed
with continuous strip of triple 0 chromic catgut to the peritoneum
and interrupted silk to the remaining layers.

Note: I should have mentioned above that a biopsy of the liver
was taken and several lymphnodes were removed from the region
of the common duct.

	3-1-05
Date reviewed	
Misc. note dictated	✓
Send ltr. to pt. from note	
Send ltr. to MD from note	
Separate letter dictated to pt.	
Separate letter dictated to MD	
OSM: ☑ SAVE	☐ THROW

SIGNATURE   R E Gross,

Michael Fayne   Age 3 months   S - 43 - 121

Material - Liver Biopsy   I.C.S.   March 27, 1943
                         #271,023

CLINICAL DATA: Jaundice since birth ? obstruction

Operation - Exploratory Laparotomy

CLINICAL DIAGNOSIS: Intrahepatic Disease with Cirrhosis

GROSS DESCRIPTION: The specimen consists of a piece of liver, which measures
1.2 x 1 x 0.4 cm. Its external surface and the cut surfaces are smooth and
greenish. The lobular markings are not prominent.

Also submitted are two lymph nodes, which together measure 1 x 0.6 x 0.4 cm.
They are greenish-gray, nodular, and firm. A piece of each tissue is fixed
in formalin.

(F.K.M.)

MICROSCOPIC: Three sections, H. & E.; two sections, Foot's Reticulum.

Two H. & E. and one Foot's reticulum show the liver biopsy. The architecture
is definitely obscured. Instead of the usual hepatic lobules in which the liver
cells form cords extending from the portal regions to the central vein, the
liver cells in these sections have no definite or regular arrangement. The
lobules are irregular. The liver cells are large, pale, swollen, and foamy.
They are frequently multinucleated. They contain considerable bile. They are
arranged in an irregular pattern with sinusoids, which are indistinct and irregular. The interlobular connective tissue is increased. The bile ducts are inconspicuous, and only a few of them can be identified as such. These are lined
by low cuboidal epithelium. The Kupffer cells are filled with bile. The blood
vessels are congested.

One H. & E. and one Foot's reticulum sections show the lymph node. The architecture is well preserved. The primary follicles are rather indistinct. They occupy
the cortical region. They show no secondary centers. The follicles are made up
of the true lymphocytes. The sinusoids also contain lymphocytes as well as many
brown pigment containing macrophages. The blood vessels are congested.

(F.K.M.)

DIAGNOSES: 1. Bile Stasis of Liver consistant with Area of Regeneration in Liver
               seat of Toxic Hepatitis
        2. Lymph Nodes - Bile Pigmentation of

Sidney Farber M.D.
Pathologist

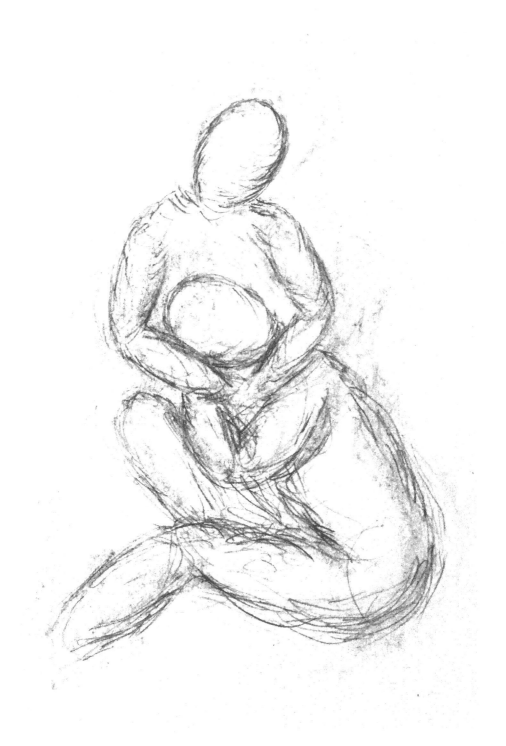